CHAIR YOGA

FOR SENIORS

Fully **Illustrated Workout Plan** for Reclaiming **Strength,**
Enhancing **Flexibility,** and Restoring **Balance**
in Just **28 Days**

FitLife Solutions – Grow Your Health

ISBN: 9798325721847

PAGE 2

Table of Contents

About the Author 4

Introduction 5

Special Bonus Offer! 7

What is Chair Yoga? 8

Benefits of Chair Yoga for Seniors 9

Chair Yoga' Safety Tips and Precautions 12

Breathing 14

What is needed for Chair Yoga? .16

Types of Exercises 17

    Warm-Ups 17

    Exercises for Hands and Shoulders 29

    Exercises for Legs and Hips 41

    Exercises for Back 48

    Full Body Exercises 57

    Exercises with Extra Weight 75

    Stretches 84

    Exercises for Arthritis 93

28-Day Workout Challenge 104

28-Day Challenge for Arthritis .109

Conclusion 111

References 112

About the Author

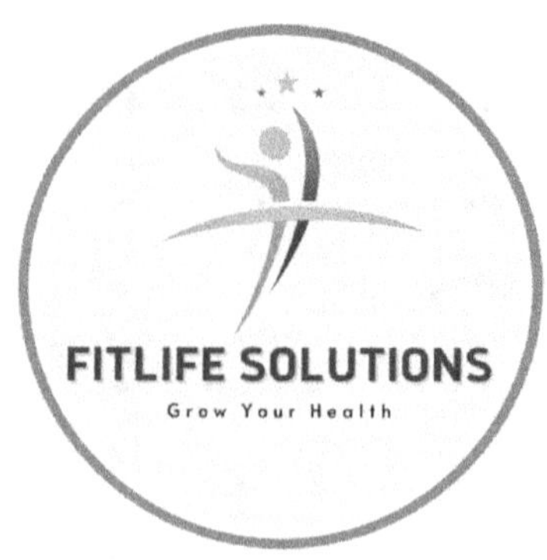

FitLife Solutions is a leading provider of fitness programs tailored to individuals of all ages and diverse needs. Our mission is to empower people to live healthier, happier lives through personalized fitness solutions.

At FitLife Solutions, we understand unique fitness goals and requirements and, therefore, offer a wide range of programs designed to cater to the specific needs of each individual. Whether you're a busy professional looking for more efficient workouts, an individual who has specialized fitness needs, or a senior wanting to improve flexibility and mobility, there's a program just for you.

Our team of certified trainers and experienced fitness experts work effortlessly to develop innovative, effective workout plans for the highest level of effectiveness, safety, and enjoyment. The latest research in exercise science is combined with practical, real-world applications when we create programs that deliver tangible results.

At FitLife Solutions, we strongly believe fitness is for everyone, regardless of ability, age, or background. We make fitness accessible, enjoyable, and rewarding for everyone, and we support you along your journey to better health and wellness.

Introduction

Welcome to the transformative world of chair yoga designed specifically for seniors. This book takes you on a journey to experience the rejuvenating power of yoga right from the comfort of your chair.

Chair yoga helps to maintain physical health, balance, flexibility, and mental well-being. It's a safe and effective way for the senior population to enhance their quality of life, reduce stress, strengthen muscles, and improve overall mobility.

This book contains a 28-day workout plan that does just that! By spending 15 minutes each day, your life will be changed. We will explore a range of seated poses, gentle stretches, breathing techniques, and relaxation practices—all designed to promote health and vitality.

In addition to a 28-day chair yoga workout plan, this book includes a supplemental joint program designed for arthritis, a frequent condition among the elderly. The arthritis program provides specific wrist exercises and techniques intended to reduce joint pain, increase range of motion, and improve overall joint health. Both programs can be launched simultaneously. So no matter if you are trying to enhance flexibility, alleviate joint stiffness, and find moments of peace, chair yoga is a complete solution.

Introduction

You are invited to come on a personal journey of discovering yourself and working toward well-being. Through this continuous practice and mindful engagement, you'll witness the transformative effects of chair yoga on your mind, body, and spirit. Together, we will navigate the path of chair yoga and embrace the joy of movement, the serenity of inner stillness, and the power of breath.

This book is so much more than a guide! So, let's start by making each day a great one. What are you waiting for? Take a seat, get comfortable, and let's start on this wonderful journey of chair yoga!

Namaste,
FitLife Solutions Team

Special Bonus Offer!

Hello Readers,

You are a valued member of our fitness community, so we're excited to offer a wonderful bonus to help you on your path to fitness! Simply scan the **QR code** or **click on the link below**, and you'll be directed to our supplementary **Workout Progress Journal.**

QR code:

or **link:** Workout Progress Journal

The journal will assist you along your way toward fitness by providing a means to track your workouts, set individual goals, and monitor the progress you are making. The easy-to-use format and comprehensively-designed journal is a great tool to keep you on track, motivated, and accountable as you reach your fitness goals.

Don't miss out on this incredible opportunity to take your fitness journey to the next level.

Happy training,
FitLife Solutions Team

What is Chair Yoga?

Chair yoga is just like it sounds. Traditional yoga poses and practices are adapted to be executed while sitting down on a chair or using a chair for support. Chair yoga is designed for everyone, especially for those individuals who may have difficulty with traditional yoga poses because of their physical limitations, mobility issues, and advanced age.

Chair yoga offers many benefits of traditional yoga: improved balance, strength, flexibility, and relaxation. It incorporates modified yoga poses, breathing techniques, relaxation exercises, and meditation while performed in a seated position. Adaptable for people of all ages and fitness levels, chair yoga is a great choice for seniors, those with disabilities, and others recovering from surgery or an injury. It is also ideal for anyone who needs the support of a chair while exercising. Chair yoga can be practiced in your home, classroom, or rehabilitative or therapeutic setting.

Another important benefit of chair yoga is its versatility. The practices and poses can be modified for the needs of each practitioner. That way, the yoga experience is accessible and personalized. Chair yoga can be easily integrated into daily routines to maximize health benefits, most notably increased range of motion, reduced stress, improved posture, and enhanced overall well-being.

The gentle nature of chair yoga provides an opportunity to connect with the body, breath, and mind in an environment that nurtures and supports while boosting overall health, vitality, and a feeling of inner peace.

Benefits of Chair Yoga for Seniors

Chair yoga offers numerous benefits for seniors and those with limited mobility. **These are some of the advantages:**

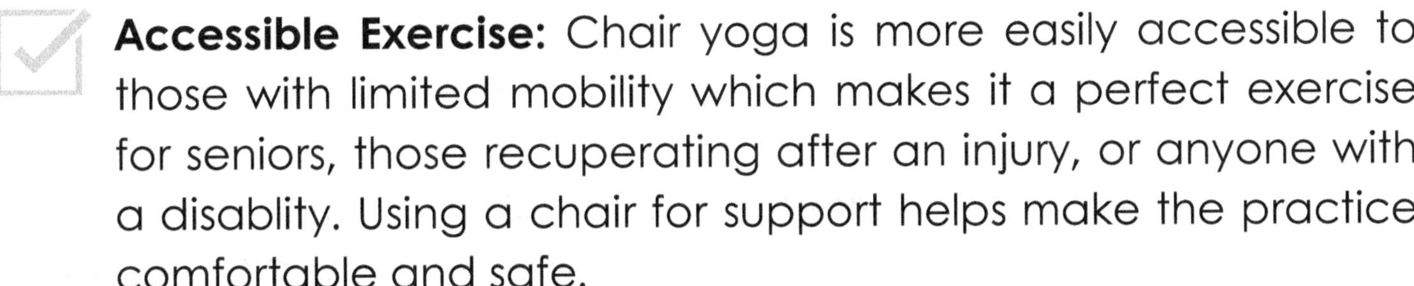 **Accessible Exercise:** Chair yoga is more easily accessible to those with limited mobility which makes it a perfect exercise for seniors, those recuperating after an injury, or anyone with a disablity. Using a chair for support helps make the practice comfortable and safe.

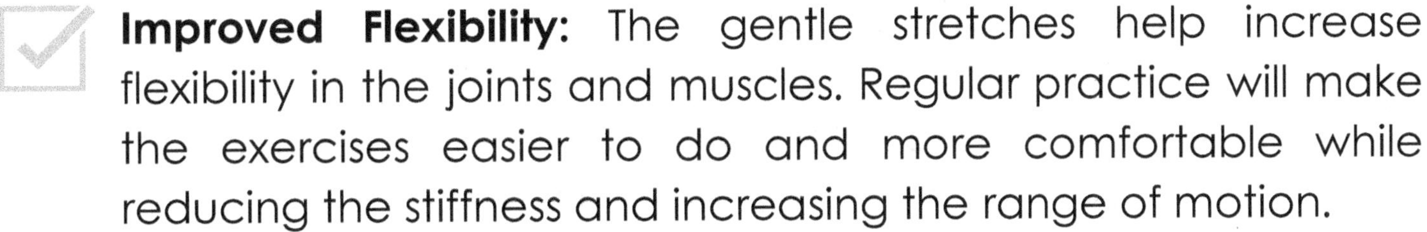 **Improved Flexibility:** The gentle stretches help increase flexibility in the joints and muscles. Regular practice will make the exercises easier to do and more comfortable while reducing the stiffness and increasing the range of motion.

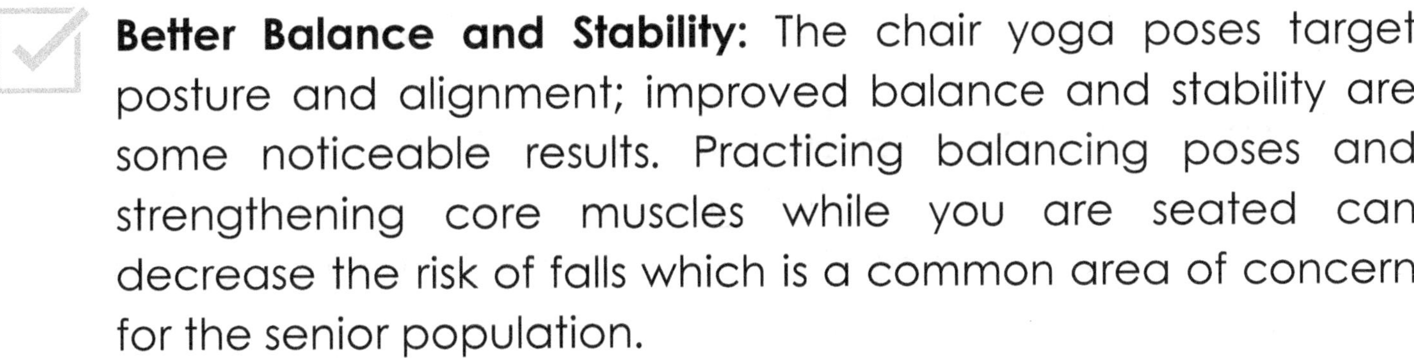 **Better Balance and Stability:** The chair yoga poses target posture and alignment; improved balance and stability are some noticeable results. Practicing balancing poses and strengthening core muscles while you are seated can decrease the risk of falls which is a common area of concern for the senior population.

Boosted Energy and Mood: Participaing in regular physical activity, including in a seated position, can boost energy levels and your general mood. Chair yoga can give you a sense of accomplishment, empowerment, and confidence, characteristics that lead to a more positive outlook on life.

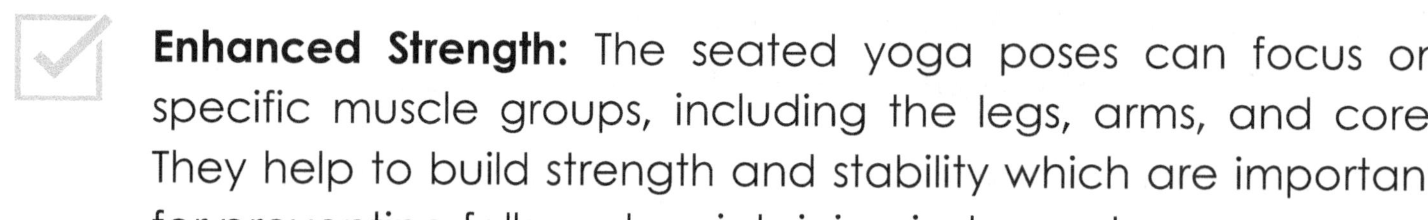

Benefits of Chair Yoga
for Seniors

✓ **Enhanced Strength:** The seated yoga poses can focus on specific muscle groups, including the legs, arms, and core. They help to build strength and stability which are important for preventing falls and maintaining independence.

✓ **Enhanced Circulation:** Several chair yoga poses can stimulate blood flow and circulation beneficial for good heart health and help prevent unwelcome conditions like edema and varicose veins.

✓ **Improved Posture:** We all know that sitting for a long time can lead to poor posture. The chair yoga exercises encourage proper alignment and spinal health which, in turn, can prevent postural issues and alleviate back pain.

✓ **Mind-Body Connection:** Chair yoga stresses body awareness and mindfulness, fostering a deeper connection between the body and mind. This, in turn, can improve overall mental clarity, focus, and concentration.

✓ **Reduced Joint Pain:** Gentle stretches and movements in chair yoga can help reduce stiffness and joint pain that comes with health-related conditions like arthritis. Additionally, daily practice can improve the lubrication of joints and reduce inflammation.

Benefits of Chair Yoga for Seniors

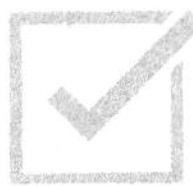 **Stress Relief and Relaxation:** Chair yoga utilizes meditation techniques and breathing exercises to promote relaxation and reduce stress levels. The process of deep breathing can calm the nervous system which leads to improved overall well-being.

Overall, chair yoga offers a and compreheansive approach to wellness, as it addresses all aspects of health: physical, mental, and emotional. It promotes self-care and encourages practioners to stay engaged and active, no matter their physical limitations.

Chair Yoga's Safety Tips and Precautions

Safety is important when practicing chair yoga, especially for individuals with physical limitations and the senior population. These are some safety tips:

- **Consult a Healthcare Professional:** 1.Before beginning the new exercise program, it's recommended to consult your doctor or healthcare provider. This is especially important for those with pre-existing health conditions. Healthcare professionals can provide guidance on whether chair yoga is appropriate for you. They will also inform you of any precautions or give further advice.

- **Adjust Your Position:** Proper alignment is the key to preventing injury. It's important to sit toward the chair's front edge. Have your feet flat on the floor, knees aligned with hips, and spine straight. The shoulders should be kept relaxed and away from your ears.

- **Modify Poses as Needed:** Chair yoga poses can be adapted to fit individual abilities and needs. If any pose causes pain or feels uncomfortable, you can modify it or skip it. Listening to your body to avoid pushing yourself beyond your limits is paramount.

- **Avoid Overexertion:** The goal is to start slowly and gradually increase the intensity of your practice and the time spent doing chair yoga. This way there will be less strain on your body or less exhaustion. You can always take a break whenever it's needed.

Chair Yoga's Safety Tips and Precautions

- **Stay Hydrated:** Drinking water before and after chair yoga practice is important for hydration. If you are exercising in a warmer environment, it's especially important.
- **Listen to Your Body:** Your body gives off signals. If a pose causes any dizziness, sharp pain, or discomfort, stop and ask a qualified instructor or healthcare professional for guidance.

Following these safety tips along with practicing mindfulness throughout the daily chair yoga sessions will allow you to reap many benefits of yoga and also minimize the risk of any injury or strain. Approaching chair yoga with patience, self-awareness, and a focus on overall well-being is important!

Breathing

Breathing, an important component of chair yoga, is necessary for promoting relaxation, reducing stress, and enhancing overall well-being. The breathing exercises in chair yoga are known as pranayama. They are integrated into the sequences and poses to foster mindfulness and deepen the mind-body connection. Let's look at how breathing is incorporated into this form of yoga.

Breath Awareness: First, chair yoga begins with an awareness of breath. You observe its natural rhythm, specifically the inhalations and exhalations without alteration or judgment.

A Coordinated Movement: The breathing is coordinated with yoga movements. The flow of energy and relaxation is enhanced through inhaling during expansive movements (e.g., reaching the arms overhead) and exhaling during contracting movements (e.g., folding forward).

Deep Breathing: Deep breathing is at the forefront of chair yoga. It is described as inhaling deeply through the nose, letting the belly expand fully, and then exhaling slowly through the mouth as the belly is drawn toward the spine. In doing so, the parasympathetic nervous system is activated which, in turn, induces a state of calm and relaxation.

Breathing

Breath Counting: Counting the breath is an integral technique to control and deepen it. Practitioners of chair yoga inhale, hold their breath, and exhale to a specific count to promote balanced, controlled breathing.

Mindful Breathing: Mindfulness of the breath is encouraged as your breath moves in and out of the body. Practitioners of chair yoga focus on the chest (rising and falling) or the belly (expanding and contracting) which anchor their awareness in the present moment.

Relaxation Techniques: Relaxation techniques that utilize the breath are incorporated in chair yoga. These techniques help to create a state of tranquility and calm. They include mindful breathing exercises, progressive muscle relaxation, and guided imagery intentionally designed to promote deep relaxation while releasing tension.

Intentional breathing techniques in chair yoga are a dynamic tool for cultivating mindfulness and inner peace while connecting with the body's innate wisdom.

What is needed for Chair Yoga?

To participate in Chair Yoga safely and effectively, you'll need to have some key items. **Specifically, you will need (a):**

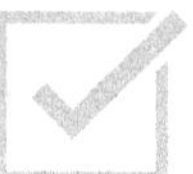 **Sturdy chair:** The chair needs to be stable and sturdy; avoid chairs with wheels, those that have legs that can slide easily on the floor, and that are too unstable and soft. A straight-backed chair without arms or supportive armrests is best.

 **Dumbbells or water bottles for substitute weights:** For exercises that need weights, you can use two 1.5-liter (6 ¼-pound) water bottles (or 1.5 kg (3.3-lb.) dumbbells if available). Feel free to adjust the weight as needed, choosing the ideal weight for your workout.

 **Comfortable clothing:** Wear clothing that stretches and is breathable, and doesn't restrict the freedom of movement. Also, avoid clothing that's too tight or too loose.

 **Water bottle:** Keep a full water bottle full nearby to help stay hydrated throughout the workout.

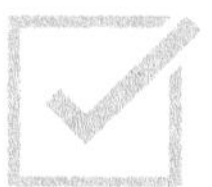 **Towel:** It's useful to have a towel to wipe away any sweat and keep your comfort level high throughout the workout.

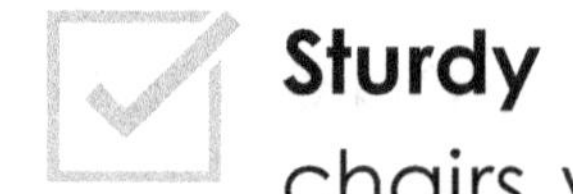 **Positive mindset:** This type of attitude and the willingness to challenge yourself increases the benefits of your exercise sessions. Listen to your body and adapt the exercises to your ability and fitness level.

Types of Exercises: Warm-Ups

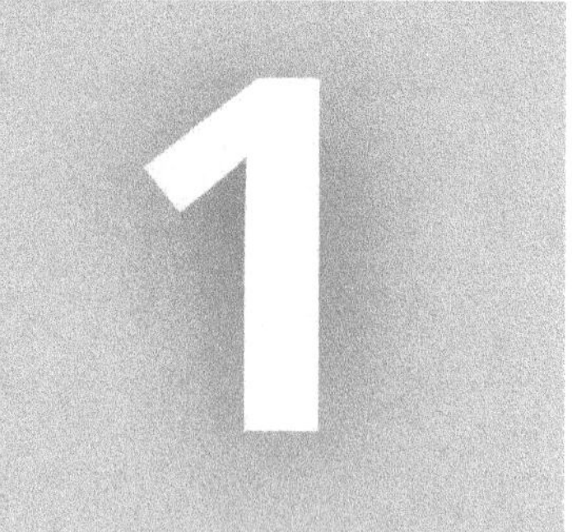

Neck Rotations

This exercise is an effective way to relieve neck tension. It also mobilizes your neck and stretches the deep neck muscles.

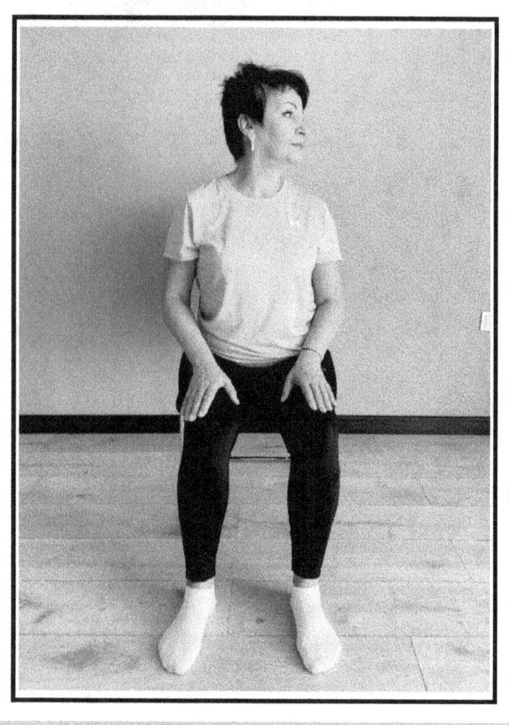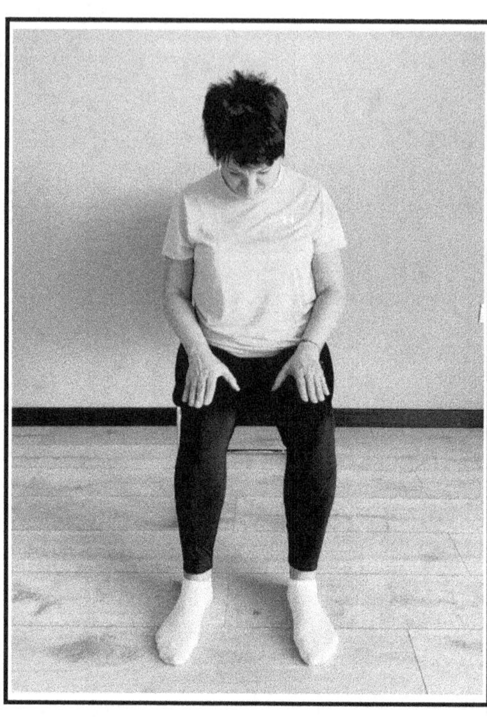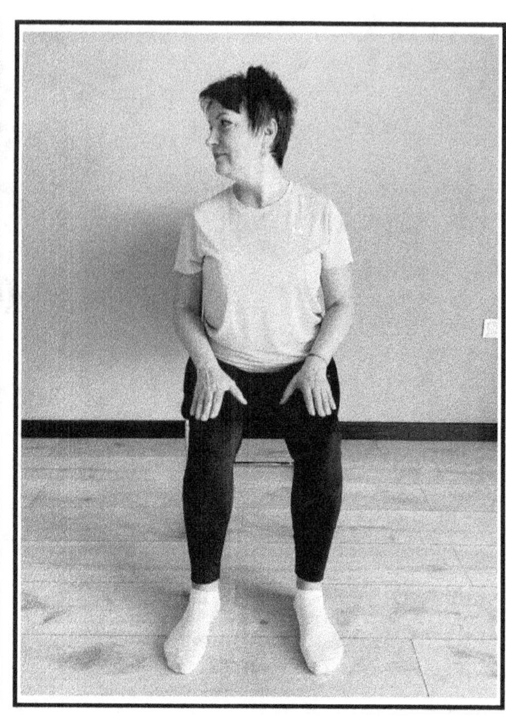

PROCEDURE:

1. Sit tall on the chair
2. Keep your knees bent
3. Put your hands on your knees
4. Gently turn your head to one side, while keeping your chin down
5. Slowly alternate between sides

SUGGESTED TIPS:

- Don't sway the head too fast
- Don't hold the breath
- Do this exercise slowly (if you sway your head too much, you'll get dizzy)

Shoulder Dancing

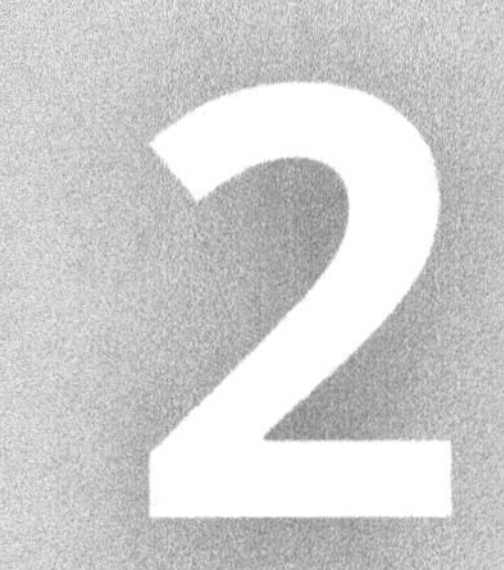

This is a fantastic exercise that warms up your shoulders, it makes your whole upper body well warmed up and relaxed.

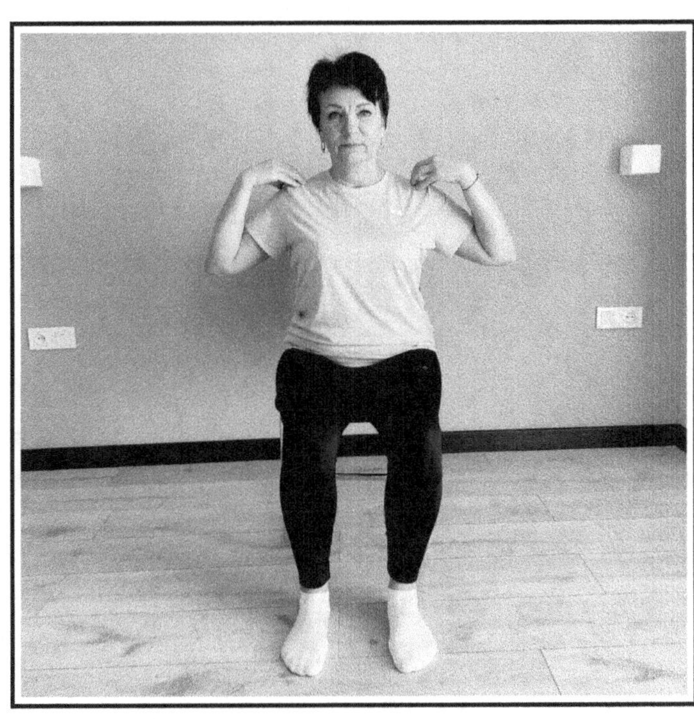 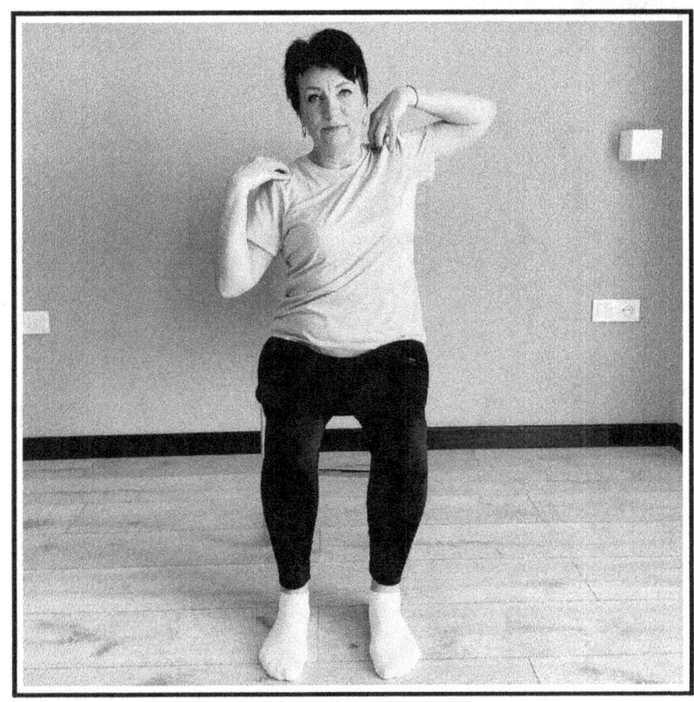

1. Sit tall on the chair
2. Keep your knees bent; put your fingers on your shoulders
3. Make a circle backward with one shoulder, and then the other shoulder
4. Make two circles back for each side and then forward
5. Repeat the exercise

- Don't hold the breath
- Don't go too fast
- Don't simultaneously do both shoulders
- Maintain regular breathing while doing this exercise

3 Shoulder Rolls

Shoulder rolls are a great exercise to relax the stiffness in the shoulders and upper trapezius.

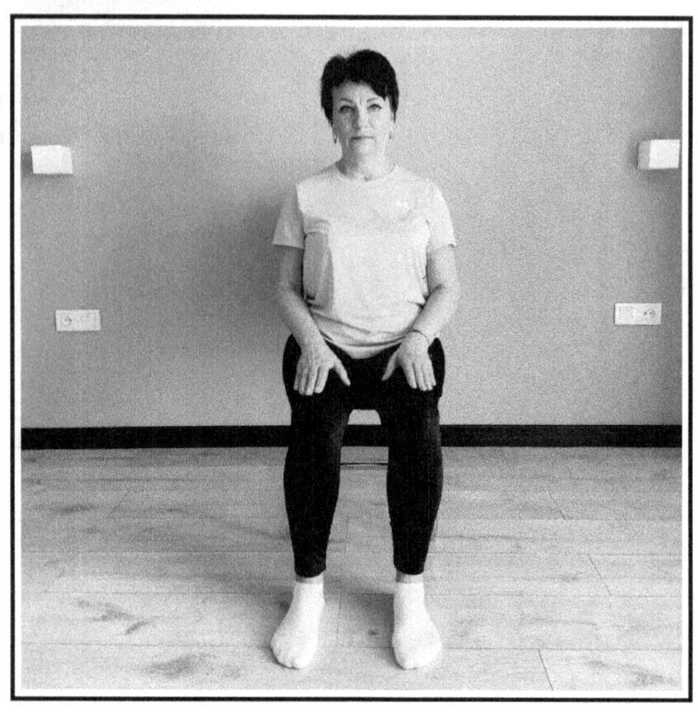 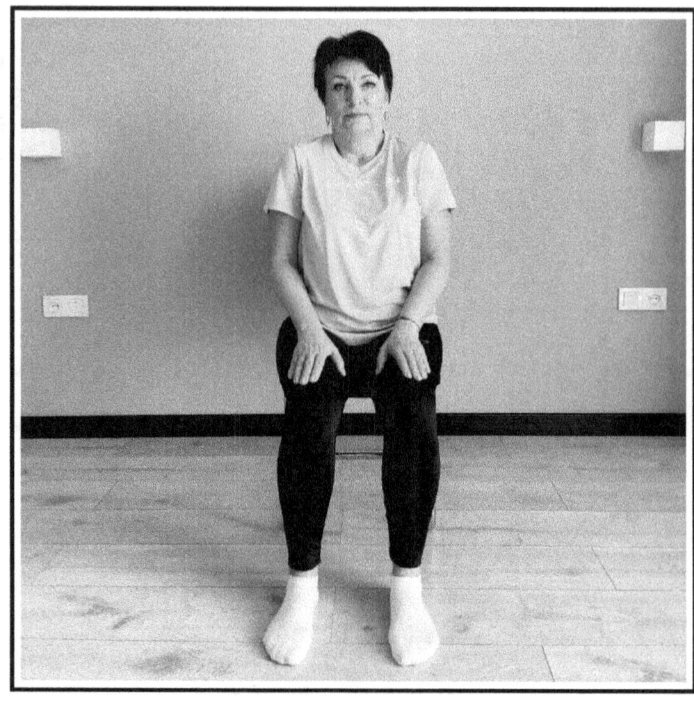

PROCEDURE:

1. Sit tall on the chair
2. Keep your knees bent
3. Put your hands on your knees
4. Roll your shoulders backward four times
5. Then, roll your shoulders forward four times
6. Repeat the exercise

SUGGESTED TIPS:

- Don't hold the breath
- Don't rush the movement
- Inhale at the beginning of the movement
- Slowly exhale as you start rolling your shoulders

Seated Crunch

This exercise is an effective way to mobilize your back and stretch your neck.

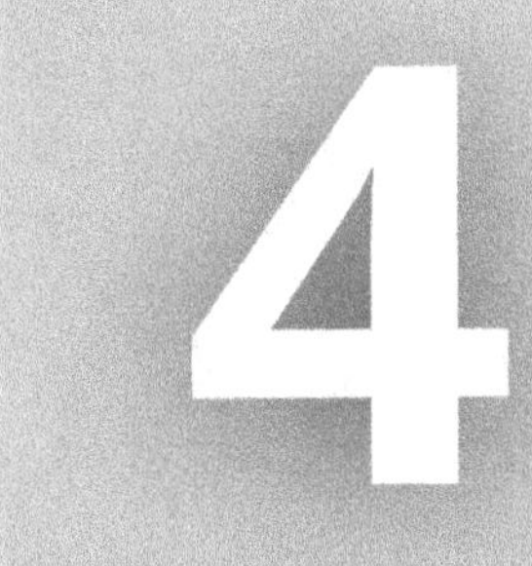

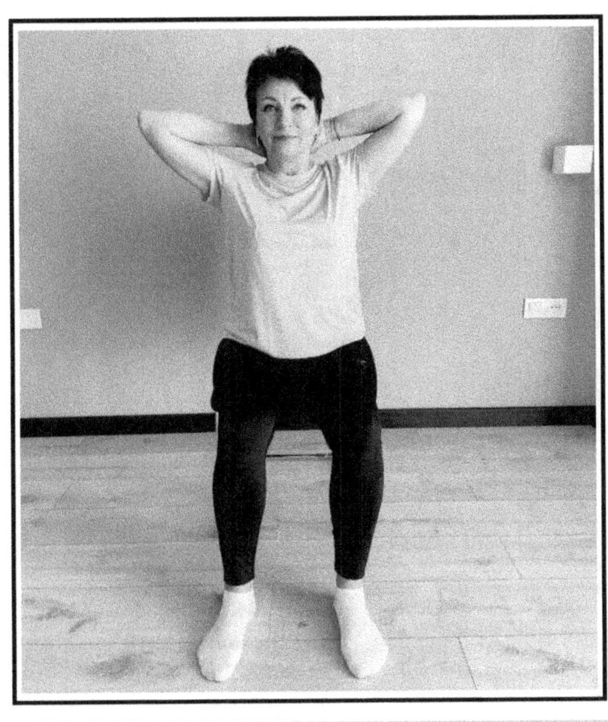

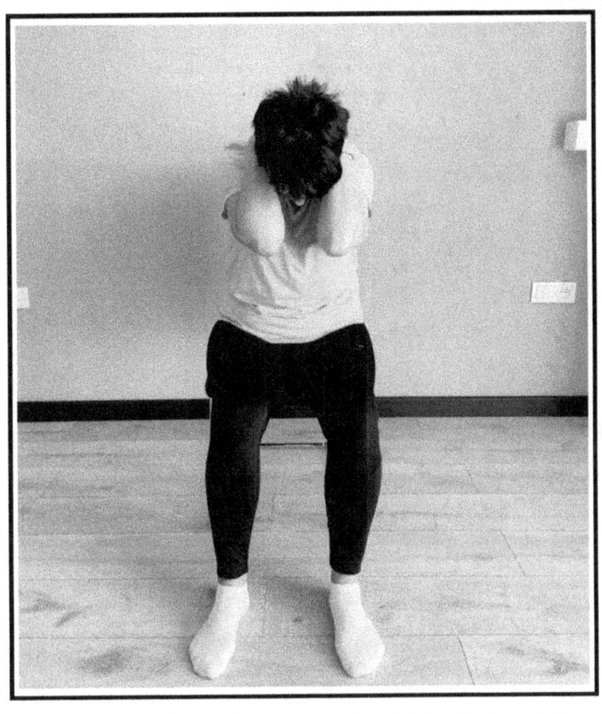

PROCEDURE:

1. Sit tall on the chair
2. Keep your knees bent
3. Put your hands behind your head
4. Bend your body and elbows toward your knee; look down
5. Extend yourself back to the previous position
6. Repeat the movement

SUGGESTED TIPS:

- Don't hold the breath
- Follow the movement with your head
- Don't go too fast
- Inhale at the beginning of the movement
- Slowly exhale as you start bending your body down

5 Arm Rotations

Arm rotations are phenomenal for improving your internal and external shoulder mobility. They're also great for warming up your shoulders.

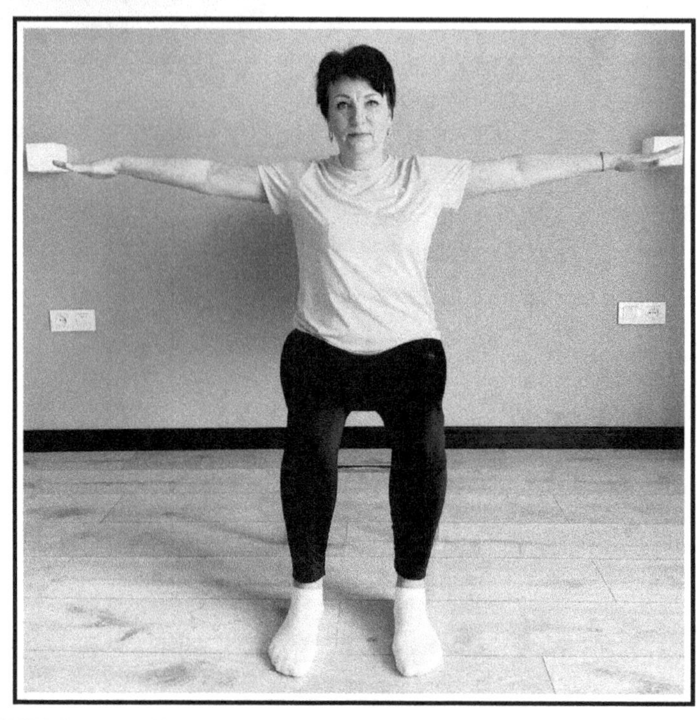 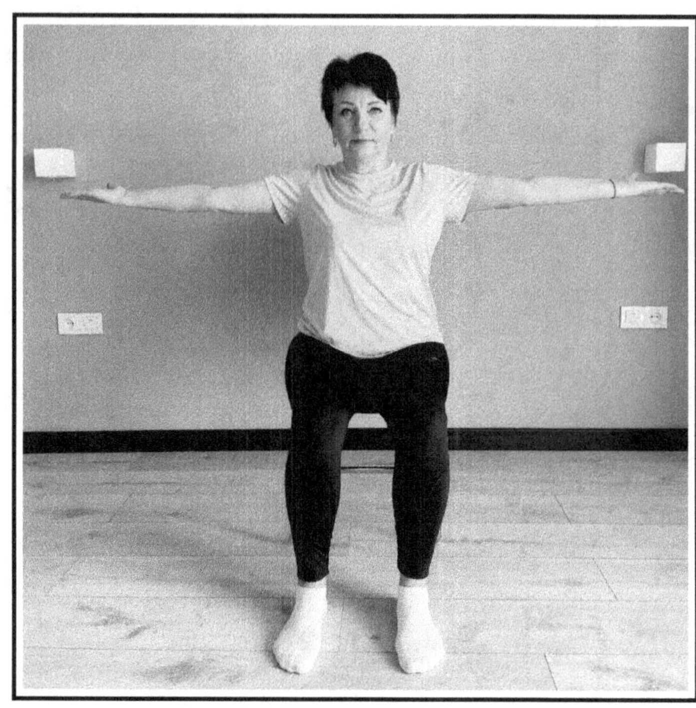

PROCEDURE:

1. Sit tall on the chair; keep your knees bent
2. Extend your arms out to the side so that your shoulders, elbows, and wrists are in line
3. Your thumbs should be facing up
4. Rotate your shoulders, elbows, and wrists inward
5. Rotate them backward to the starting position
6. Repeat the exercise

SUGGESTED TIPS:

- Don't hold the breath
- Don't rotate too fast
- Don't bend the arms
- Maintain regular breathing while doing this exercise

Arms Circles

Arm Circles are a fantastic exercise that warms up your shoulders.

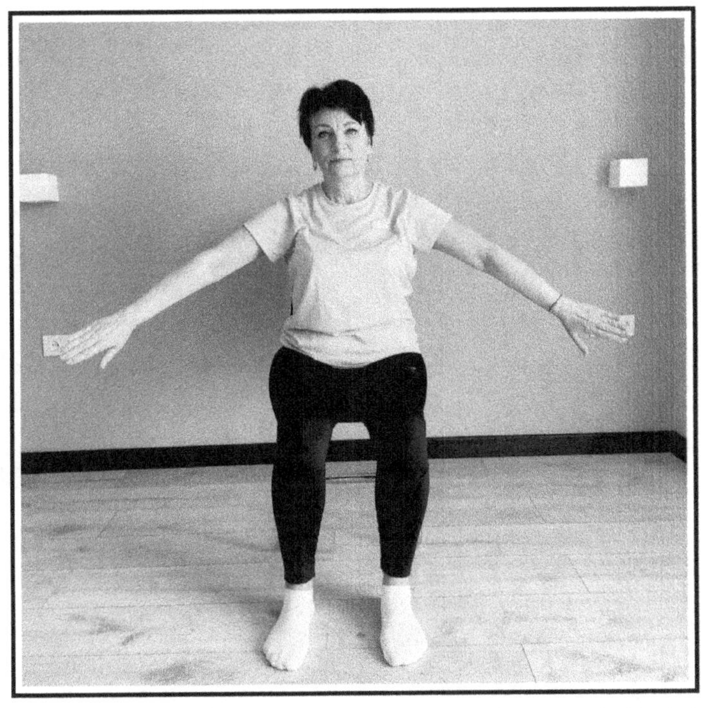 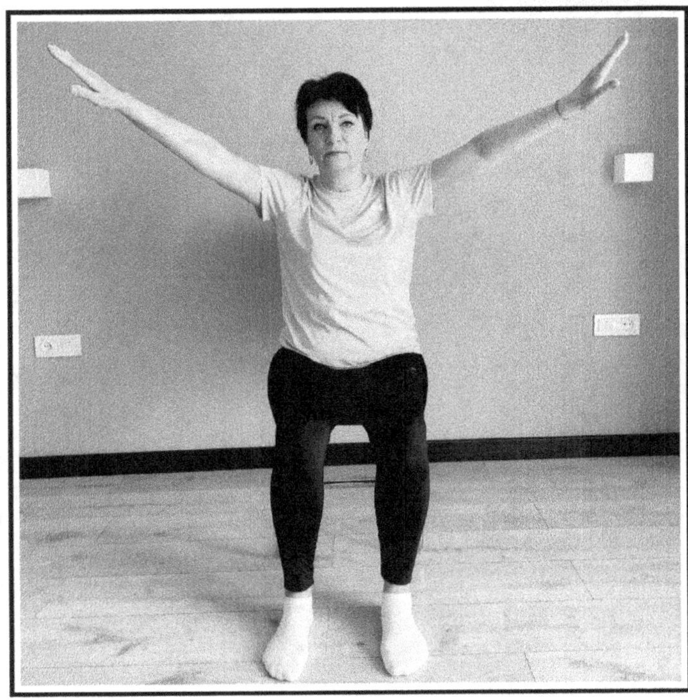

PROCEDURE:

1. Sit tall on the chair
2. Keep your knees bent
3. Lift and extend your arms out to the side at your shoulder level
4. Your wrists, elbows, and shoulders should be in line
5. Start making small circles with your shoulders
6. Alternate between going forward (three circles) and backward (three circles)

SUGGESTED TIPS:

- Don't forget to alternate between arms
- Don't bend the elbows
- Don't hold the breath
- Maintain regular breathing while doing this exercise

Seated Shoulder Mobility

As it name says, this exercise works on your internal and external shoulder mobility.

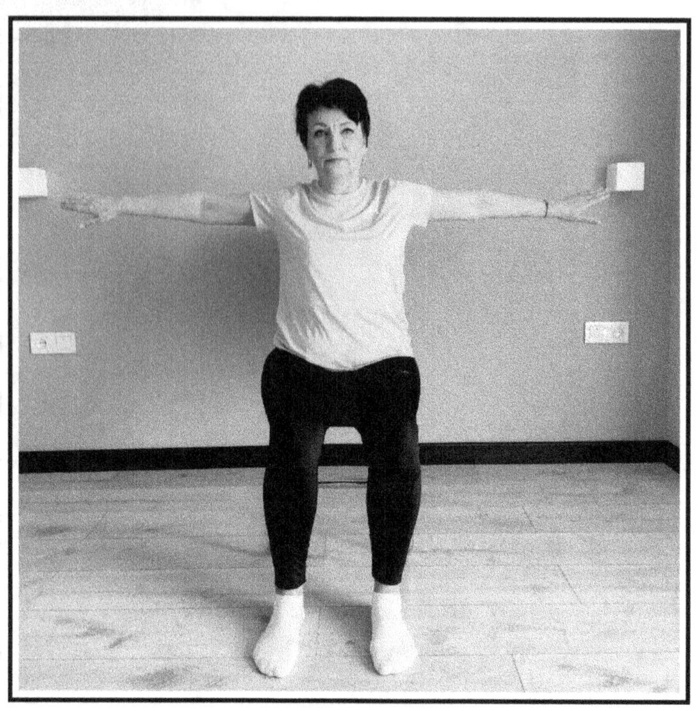 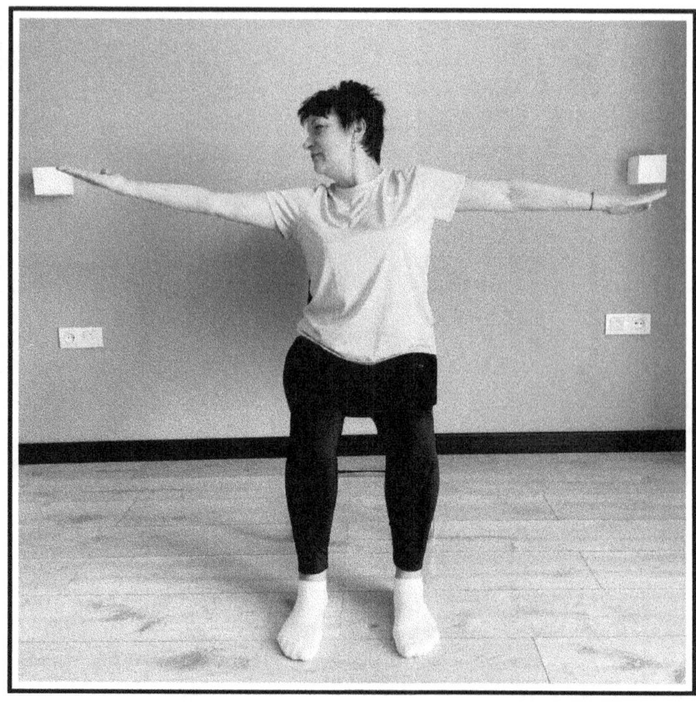

PROCEDURE:

1. Sit on the chair with your posture tall
2. Extend your arms out to the side
3. Rotate your right hand up and your left hand down
4. Look at the hand that's going up
5. Alternate between sides

SUGGESTED TIPS:

- Don't rush the movement
- Hold each rotation for a couple of seconds

Chest Opening

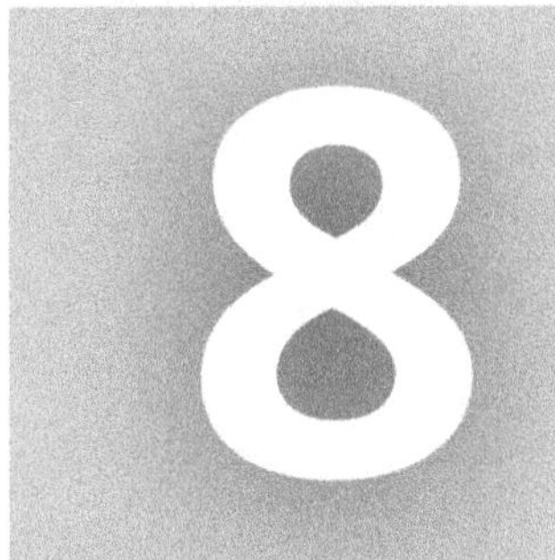

Chest Opening dynamically stretches your chest muscles. It improves your breathing.

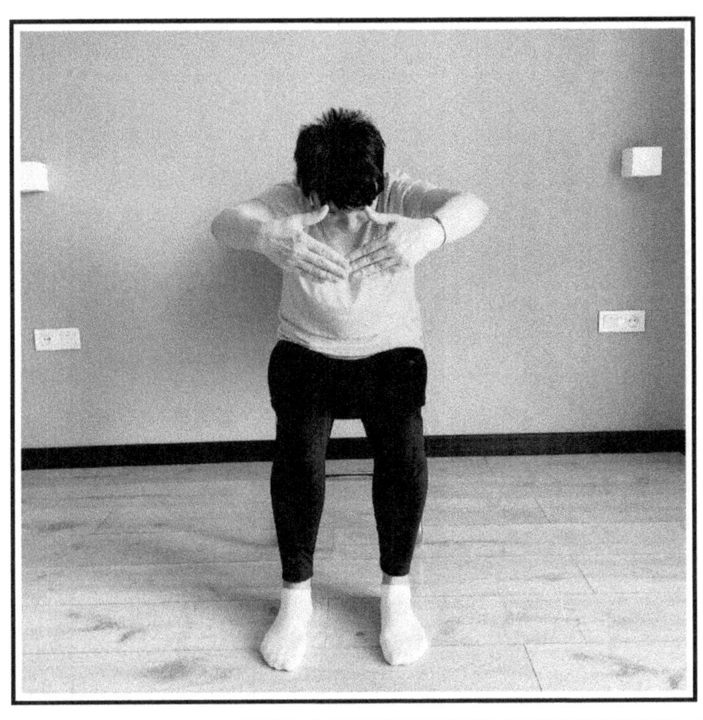
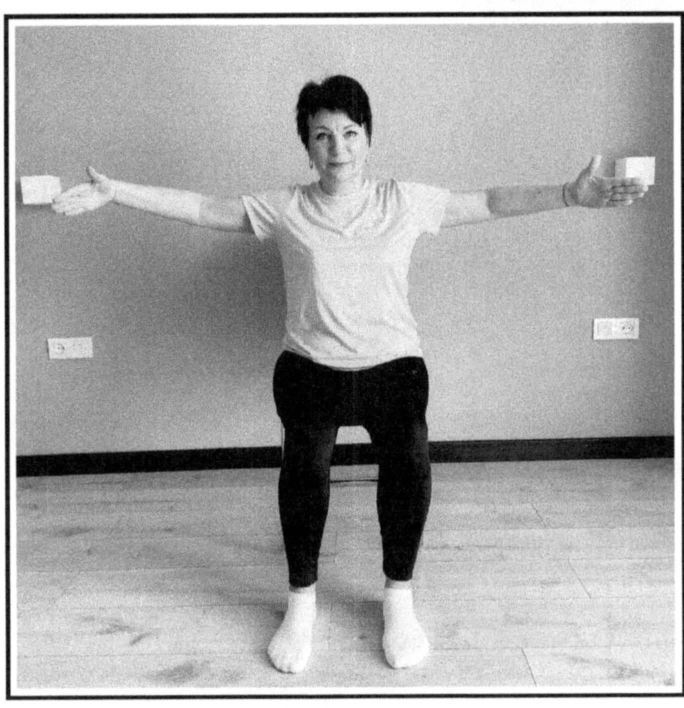

PROCEDURE:

1. Sit tall on the chair
2. Keep your knees bent
3. Extend your arms out forward, put your fingertips together; inhale
4. From that position, while keeping your elbows extended, bring them backward and push your chest out
5. Exhale and go back to the previous position
6. Repeat the exercise

SUGGESTED TIPS:

- Don't hold the breath
- Don't bend the spine
- Don't rush performing the exercise
- Take your time and do the exercise with maximum control

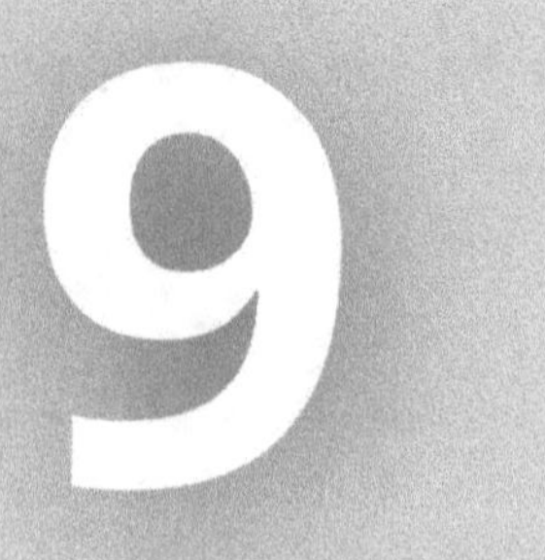

9 Hip Circles (Right, Left)

Hip circles are a fantastic exercise to improve your hip mobility.

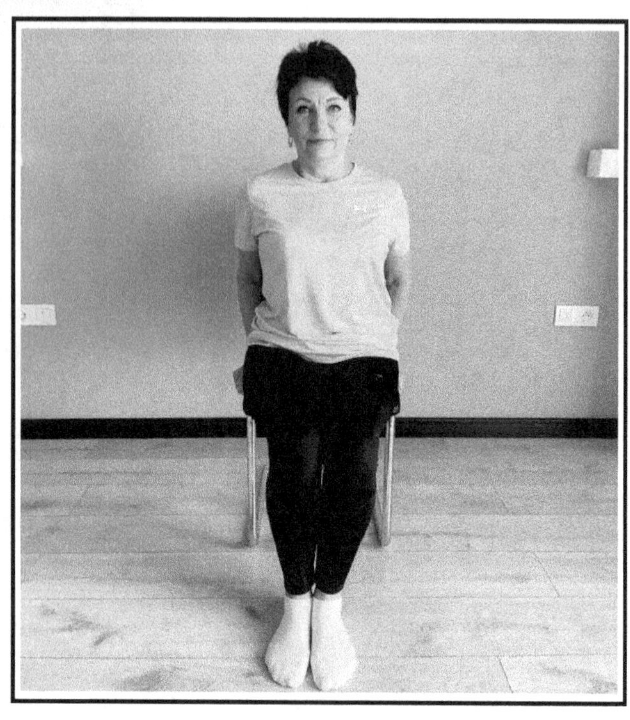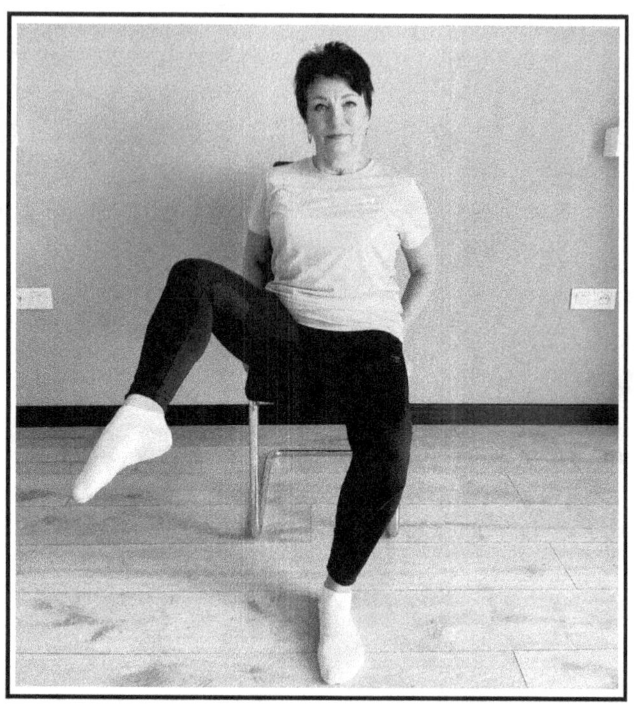

PROCEDURE:

1. Sit tall on the chair, bringing your body forward a little
2. Hold the sides of the chair with your hands
3. Lift your right leg, from the hip
4. Do two clockwise hip circles
5. Do two counterclockwise hip circles
6. Repeat the exercise
7. Perform the exercise with the left leg

SUGGESTED TIPS:

- Don't sit too far back in the chair
- Don't hold the breath
- Don't go too fast
- Inhale before you start making hip circles
- Slowly exhale when you do them

Knee Circles (Right, Left)

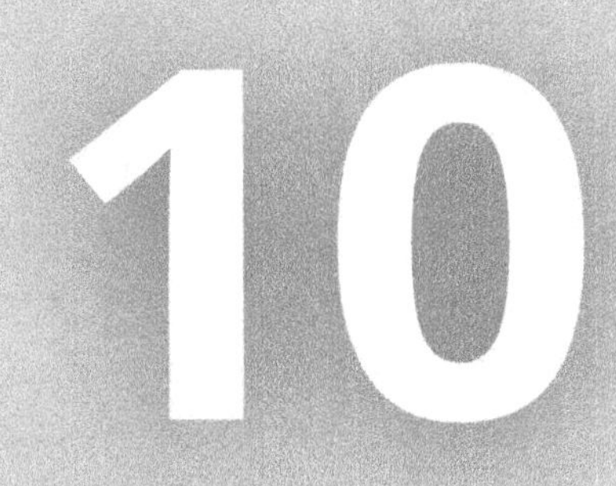

This exercise is a good warm-up exercise. It warms up your knees.

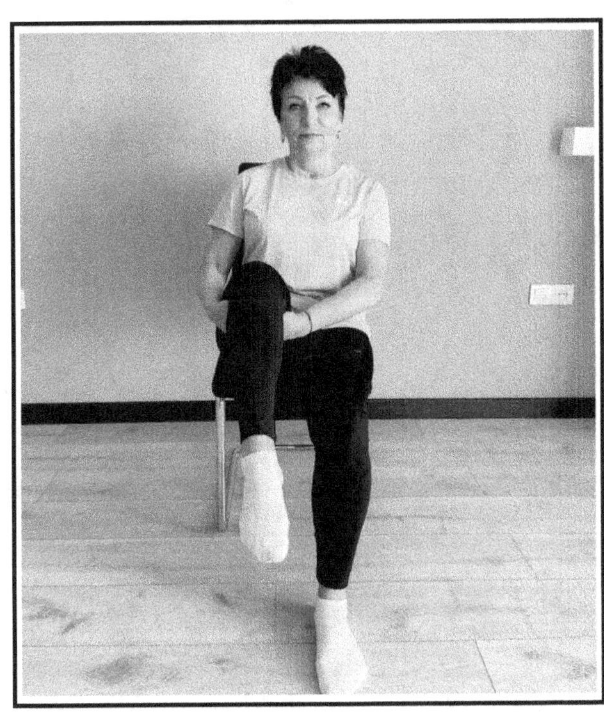 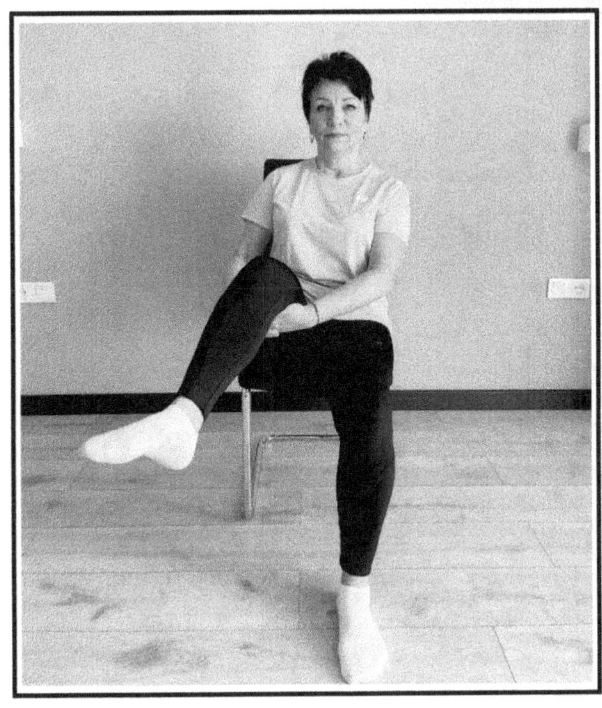

PROCEDURE:

1. Sit tall on the chair with bent knees
2. Grab your right leg with both hands and lift it
3. Make two circles with your leg clockwise, then do counterclockwise
4. Repeat the exercise
5. Perform the same exercise with the left leg

SUGGESTED TIPS:

- Don't bend the spine
- Don't hold the breath
- Don't do circles too fast
- Don't rush the exercise
- Make sure to do knee circles with full control

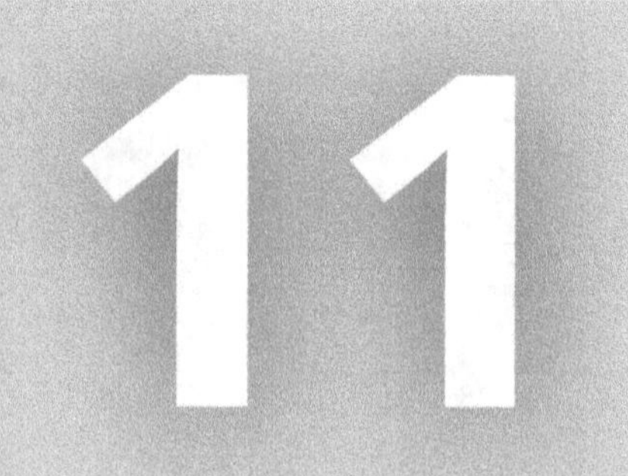

Seated Walking

This exercise strengthens your hip flexor muscles.

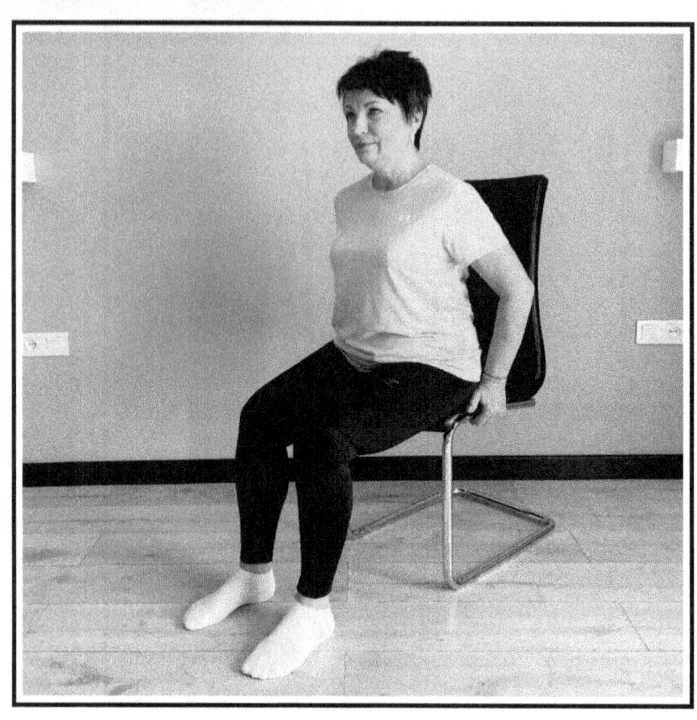 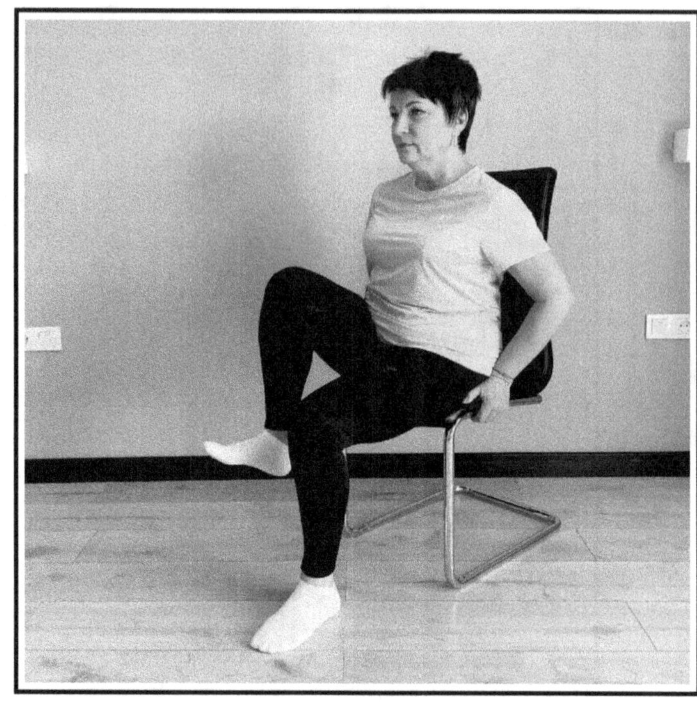

1. Sit tall on the chair with your lower back touching the chair
2. Hold the chair to the sides with your hands; inhale
3. Lift your left knee up
4. Bring the left knee down; lift your right knee up
5. Repeat the exercise alternating between legs

- Don't hold the breath
- Don't go too fast
- Don't worry about how high you're lifting your knees up
- Use any range of motion that you can

Foot Rotation Outward
(Right, Left)

This exercise works your side calf muscles.
It also improves your ankle mobility.

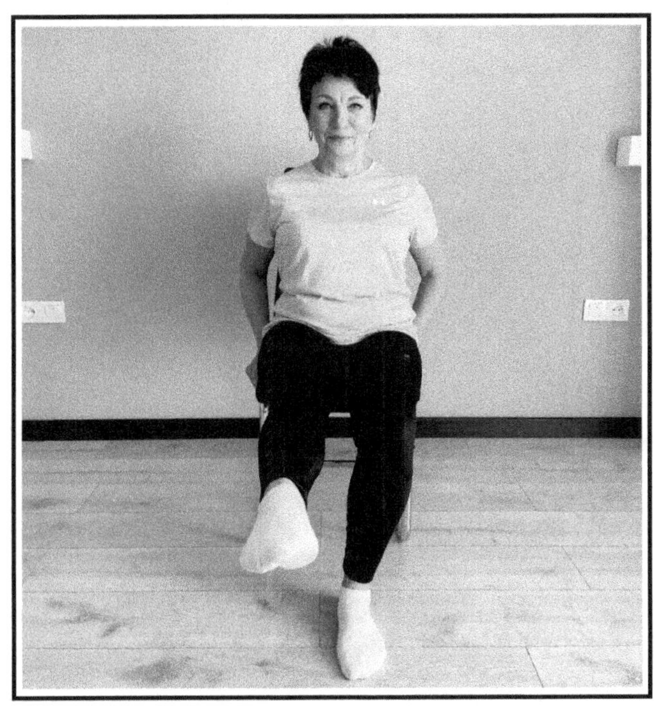 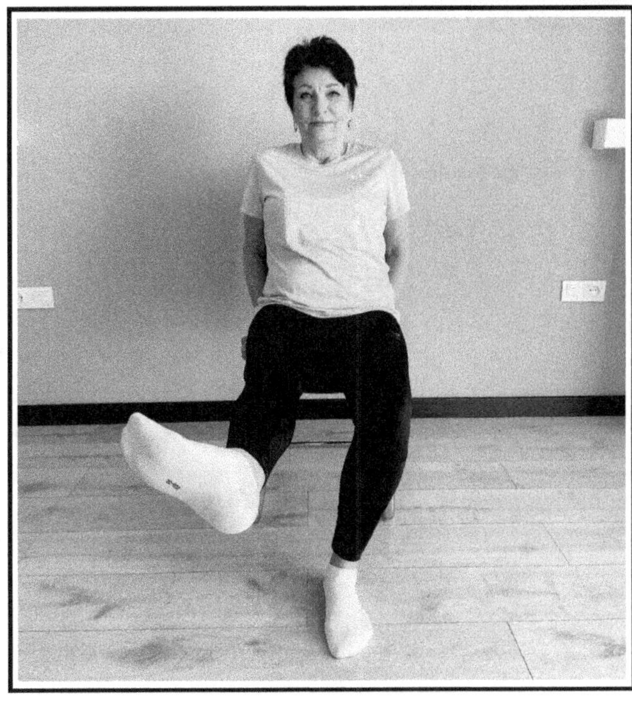

PROCEDURE:

1. Sit tall on the chair with bent knees
2. Lift and extend your right leg
3. Rotate your right foot outward
4. Repeat the movement
5. Perform the exercise with the left leg

SUGGESTED TIPS:

- Don't rotate from the hip
- Don't hold the breath
- Don't rush the movement
- Think about your pinky toe going sideways to help with outward rotation

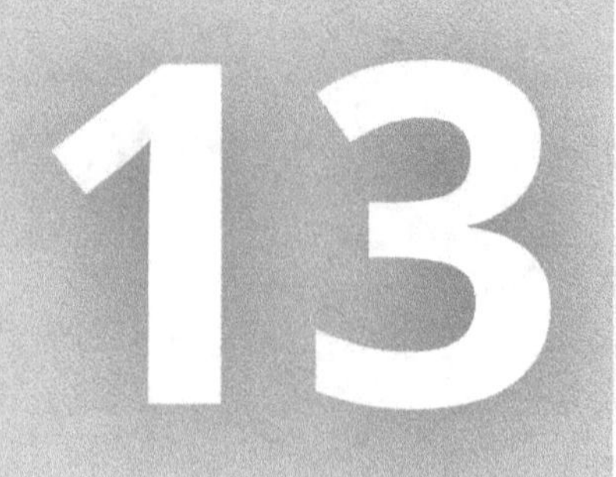

13 Foot Rotation Inward
(Right, Left)

This exercise stretches your side calf muscles. It also improves your ankle mobility.

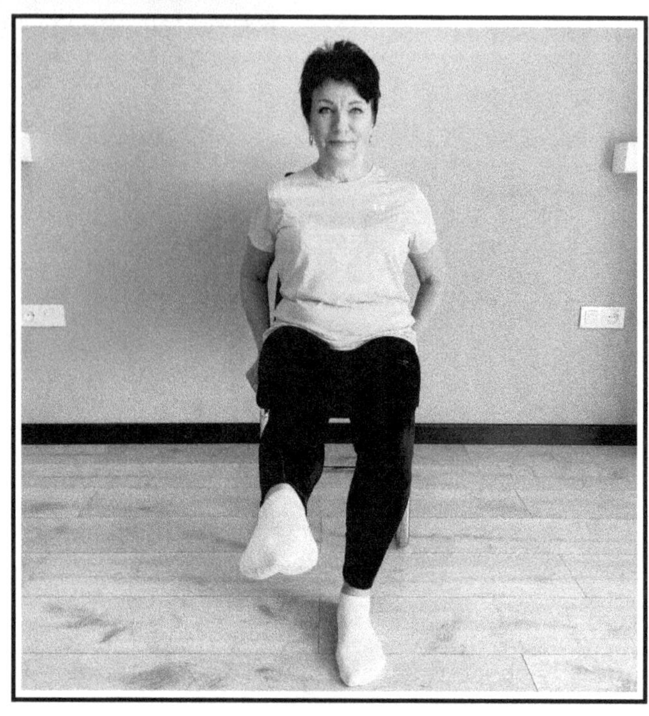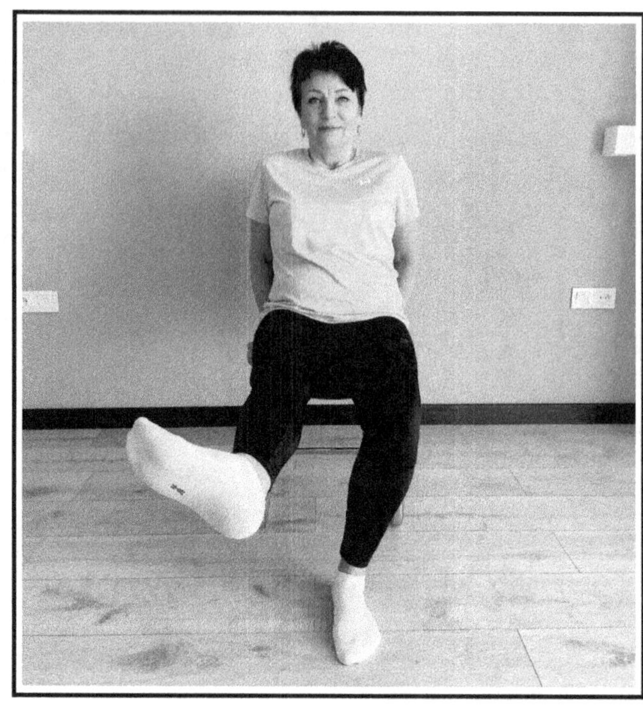

PROCEDURE:

1. Sit tall on the chair with bent knees
2. Lift and extend your right leg
3. Rotate your right foot inward
4. Repeat the movement
5. Perform the exercise with the left leg

SUGGESTED TIPS:

- Don't move the whole leg inward
- Don't rush the movement
- Don't hold the breath
- Follow the tempo of this exercise (i.e., medium – not too fast or too slow)

Exercises for Hands and Shoulders

14 Ceiling Punches

This exercise activates your triceps and shoulders. It also warms up your elbows.

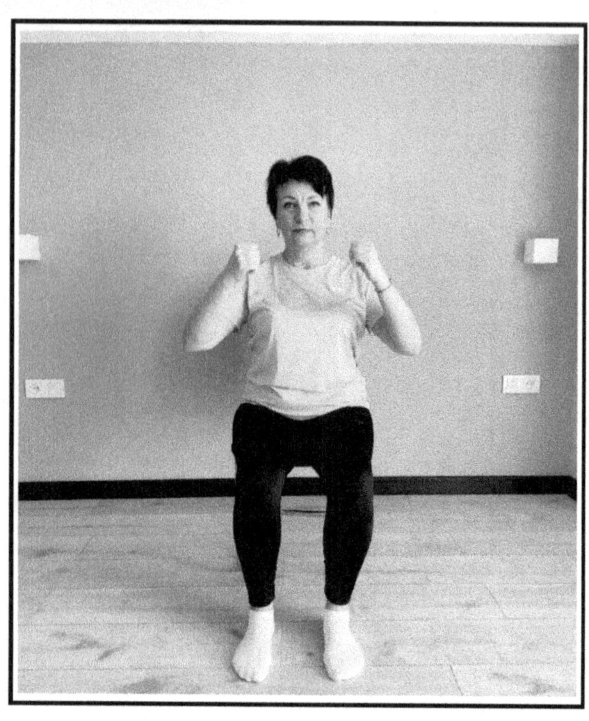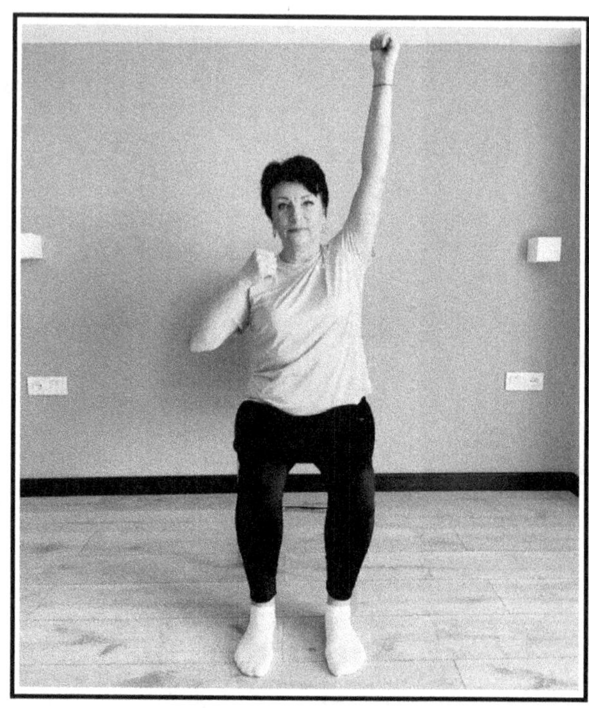

PROCEDURE:

1. Sit tall on the chair
2. Keep your knees bent
3. Bring your fists to your shoulder level
4. Extend one arm up
5. Bring it down and extend the other arm up
6. Keep alternating between sides

SUGGESTED TIPS:

- Don't hold the breath
- Don't go too fast
- Maintain regular breathing and control while doing this exercise

Underarm Pulls

Underarm Pulls are a fantastic exercise that warms up your shoulders and upper back muscles.

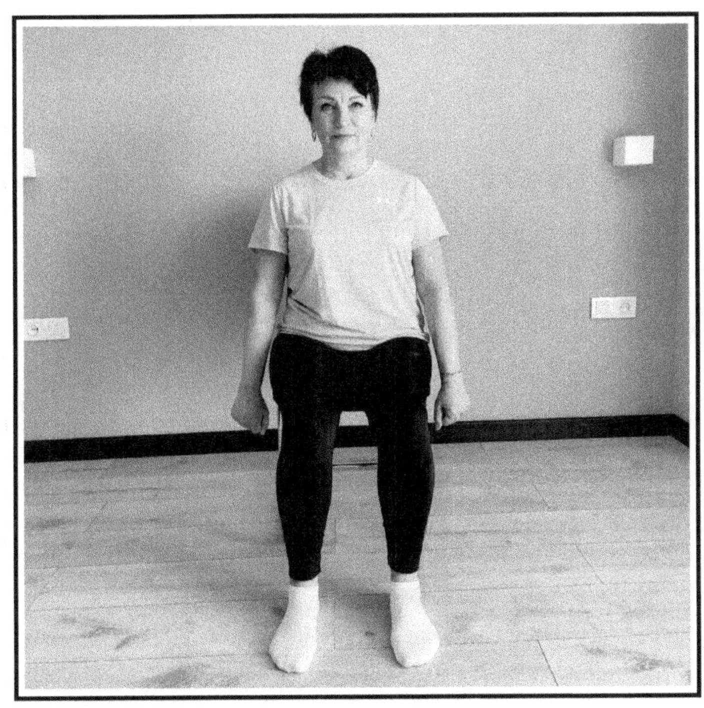
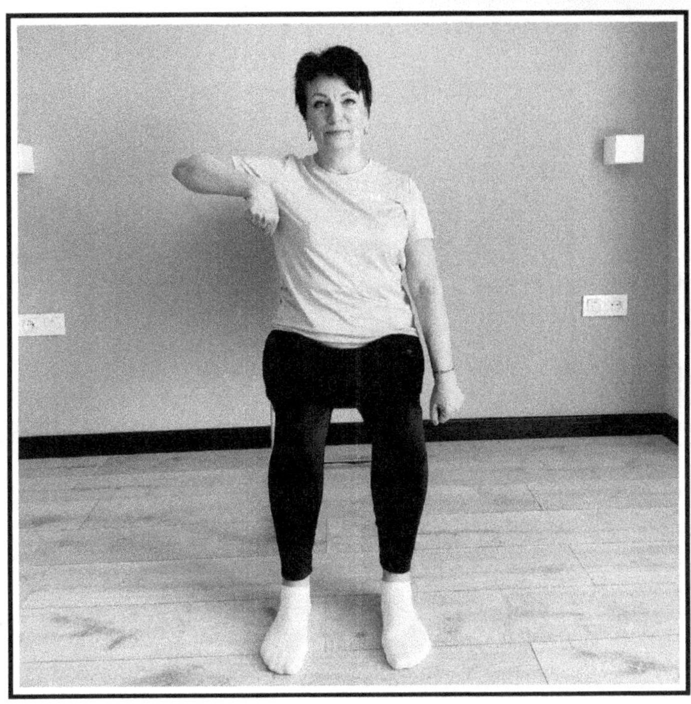

PROCEDURE:

1. Sit tall on the chair with your hands next to your sides
2. Keep your knees bent
3. Pull one hand up, close to your armpit
4. Bring it down and pull the other hand up the same way
5. Alternate between sides

SUGGESTED TIPS:

- Don't hold the breath
- Don't rush through the exercise
- Maintain regular breathing and control while doing this exercise

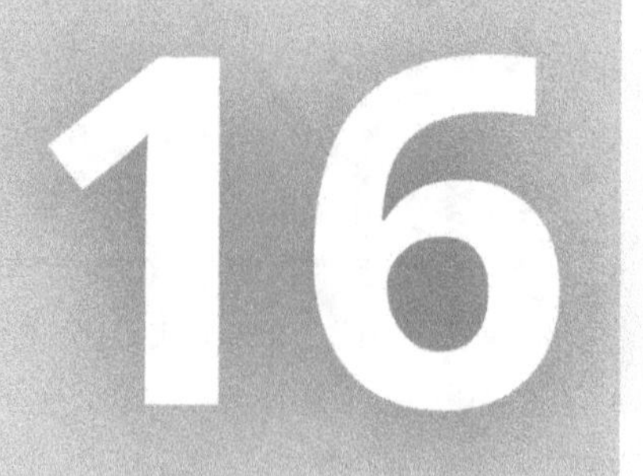

16 Air Punches

Air punches work your torso and spinal flexibility. They activate your shoulder muscles as well.

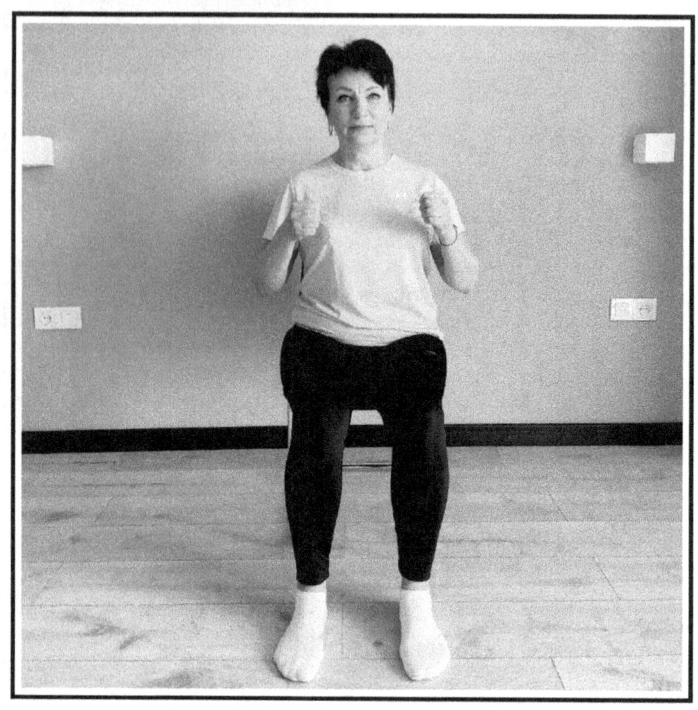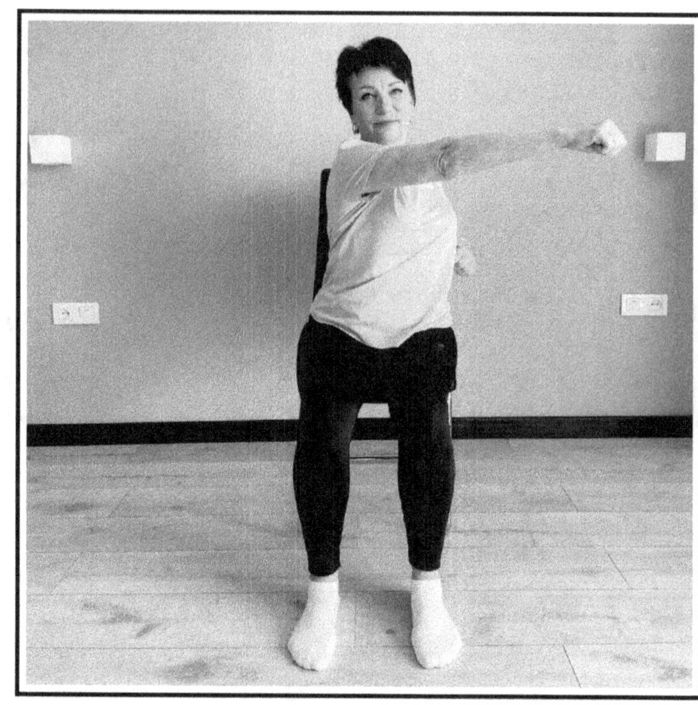

PROCEDURE:

1. Sit tall on the chair and engage your stomach
2. Keep your elbows bent by your sides, make a fist, and inhale
3. On exhale, punch toward your left side with your right hand
4. Alternate between sides

SUGGESTED TIPS:

- Don't hold the breath
- Don't go too fast
- Maintain regular breathing while doing this exercise

Bow and Arrow

This exercise activates your triceps and shoulders.
It also warms up your elbows.

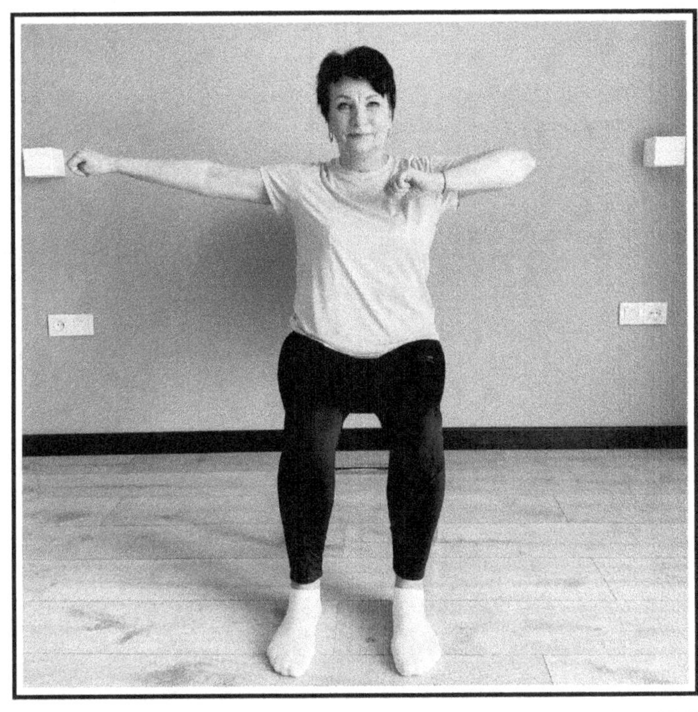 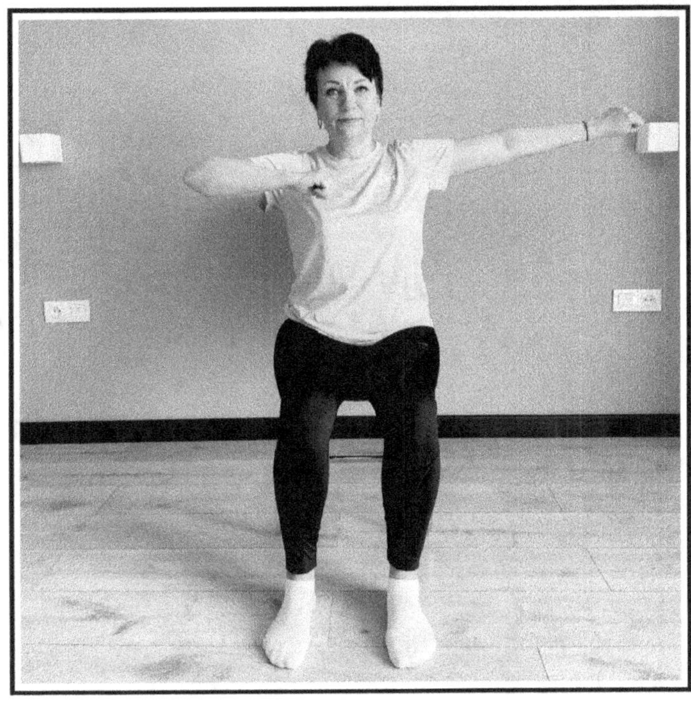

PROCEDURE:

1. Sit tall on the chair
2. Keep your knees bent
3. Bring your fists to your chest level
4. Keep your elbows bent
5. Extend one arm to the side
6. Bring it down and extend the other arm to the side
7. Alternate between sides

SUGGESTED TIPS:

- Don't go too fast
- Don't hold the breath
- Don't rush
- Maintain regular breathing and control while doing this exercise

18 Chest Flies

This is a good exercise that activates your chest muscles. It works your shoulder muscles.

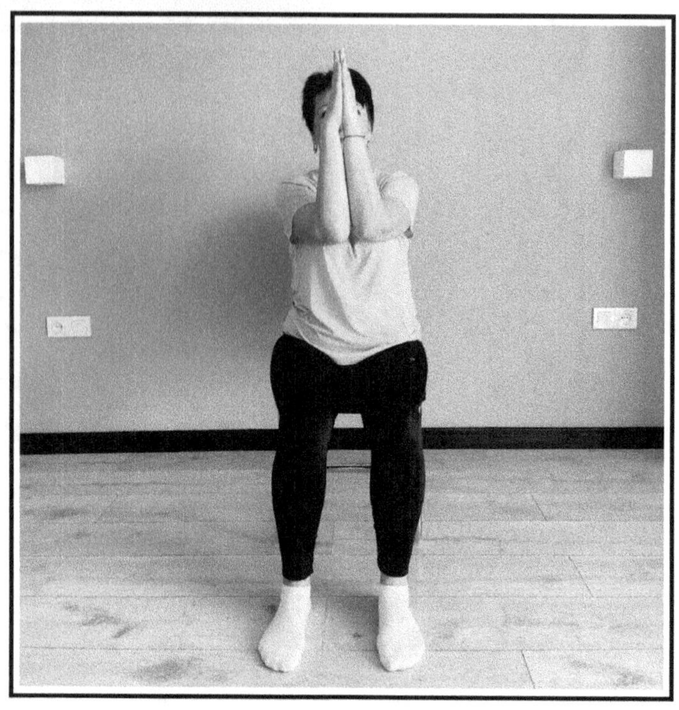 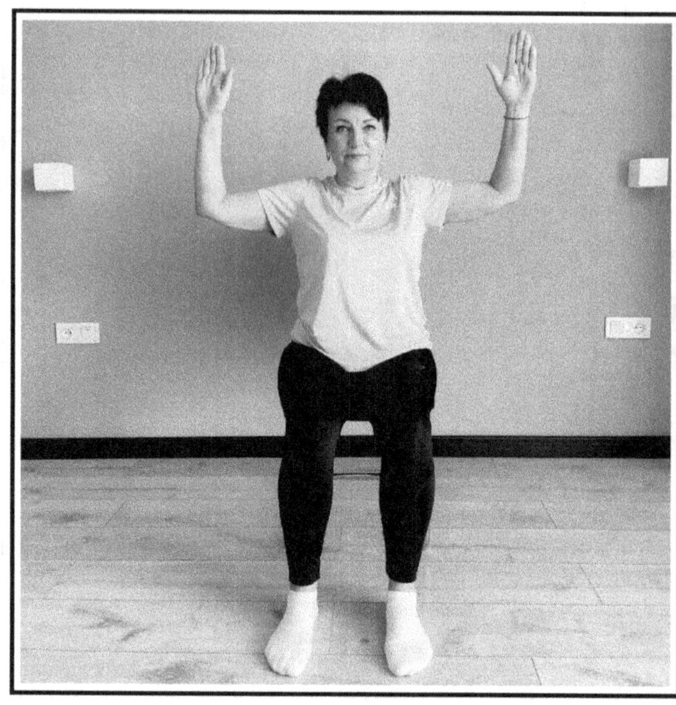

PROCEDURE:

1. Sit tall on the chair
2. Keep your knees bent
3. Put your hands up, and keep your elbows bent at a 90-degree angle
4. From this position, bring your hands and forearms together
5. Go to the previous position, repeat the movement

SUGGESTED TIPS:

- Don't rush the movement
- Don't hold the breath
- Don't arch the spine
- Inhale at the start of the movement

Arm Wipers

Arm Wipers are a fantastic exercise to warm up your shoulder, bicep, and tricep muscles.

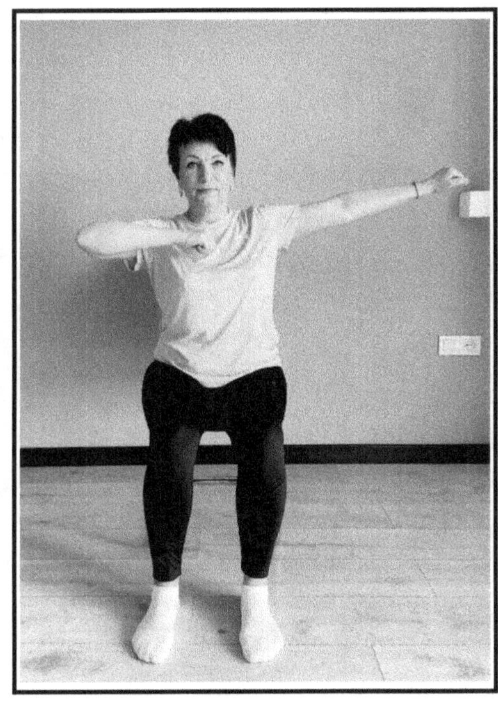 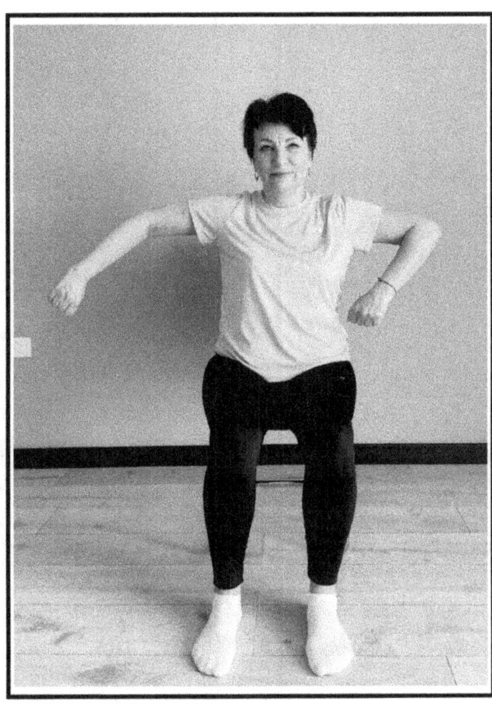 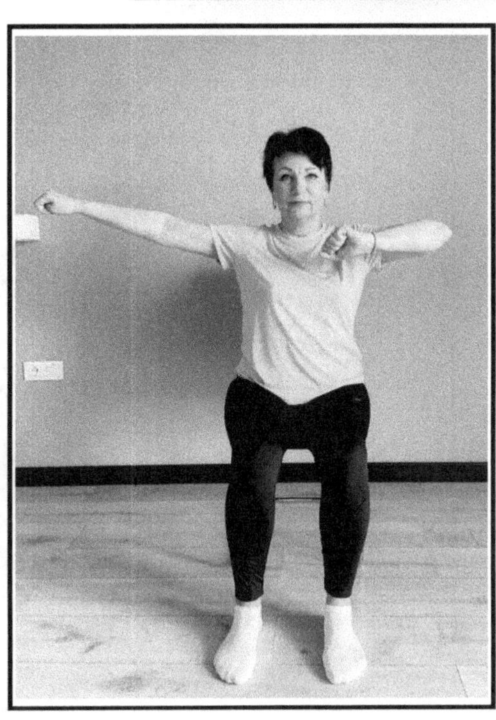

PROCEDURE:

1. Sit tall on the chair
2. Keep your knees bent
3. Extend your arms out to the side so that your shoulders, elbows, and wrists are in line
4. Bend one arm through the bottom of the other while keeping the other one extended
5. Alternate between sides

SUGGESTED TIPS:

- Don't rush the movement
- Don't hold the breath
- Maintain regular breathing while doing this exercise

Cactus Rotations

Cactus Rotations warm up and strengthen your rotator cuff muscles. They improve your internal and external shoulder mobility.

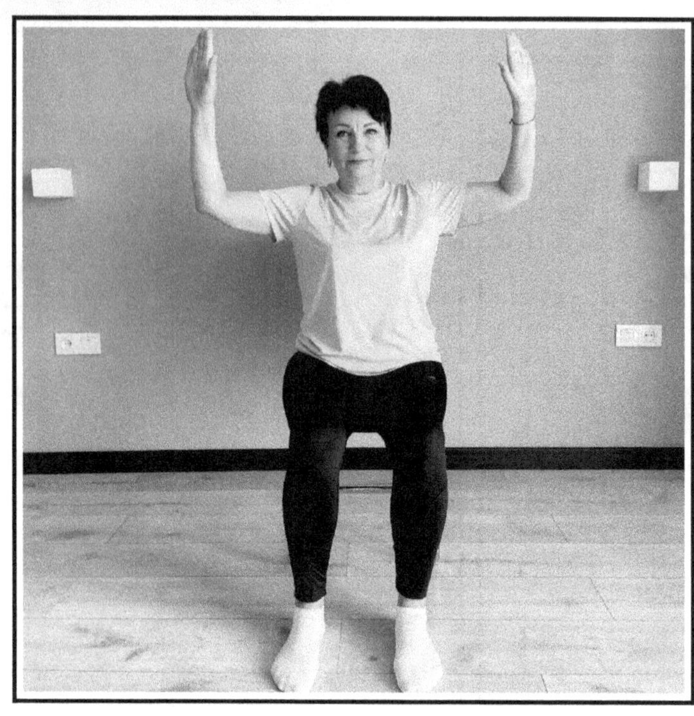

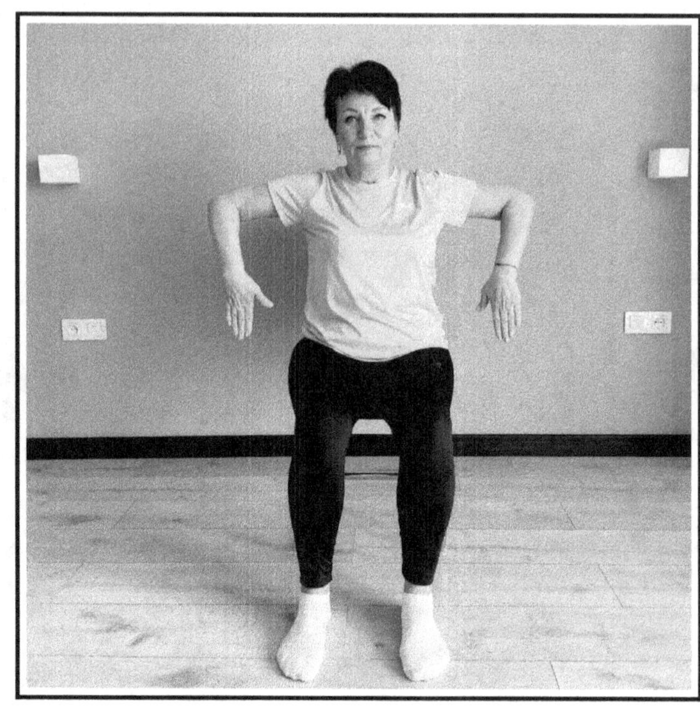

PROCEDURE:

1. Sit tall on the chair; keep your knees bent
2. Lift your arms up at a 90-degree angle
3. Without shrugging your shoulders, slowly start lowering your palms
4. Go down as far as comfortable
5. From there, slowly start bringing your palms backward as far as comfortable
6. Repeat the exercise

SUGGESTED TIPS:

- Don't go too fast
- Don't hold the breath
- Don't go to a painful range of motion
- Use full control throughout the exercise (your rotator cuffs will get the most out of the workout)

Cactus Arm Raises

This is a phenomenal exercise that works on strengthening your shoulder and rotator cuff mobility.

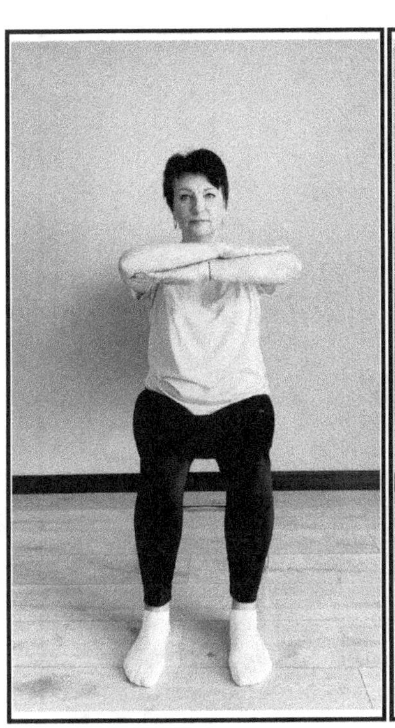 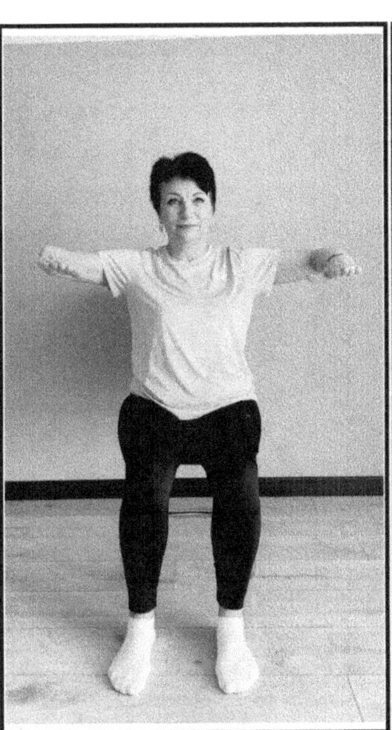 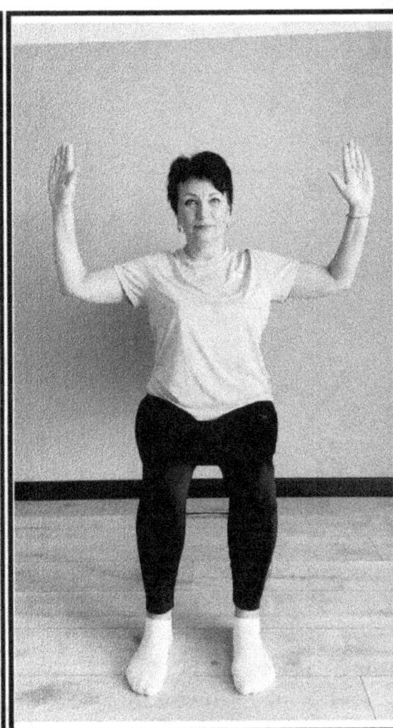 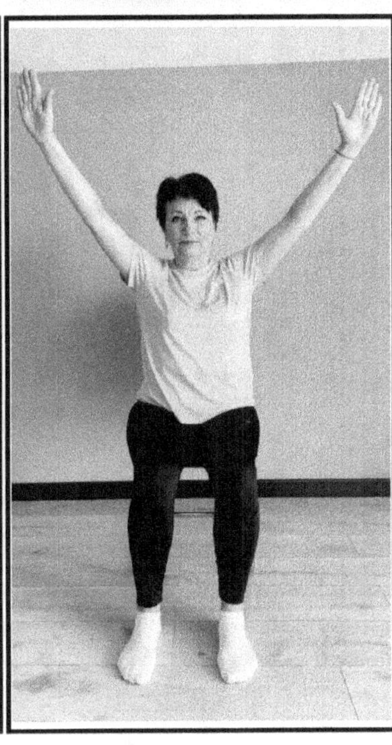

PROCEDURE:

1. Sit tall on the chair and engage your stomach
2. Keep your knees bent
3. Bend your elbows on top of each other at your chest level
4. Separate your elbows and bring them backward
5. Rotate your hands up
6. Press up from that position
7. Go to initial position; repeat the exercise

SUGGESTED TIPS:

- Don't hold the breath
- Don't rush through the exercise
- Take your time and do the exercise slowly with maximum control
- Maintain regular breathing
- Be careful to avoid feeling any joint pain

Arm Extensions (Right, Left)

Arm extensions mobilize your shoulders and elbows.

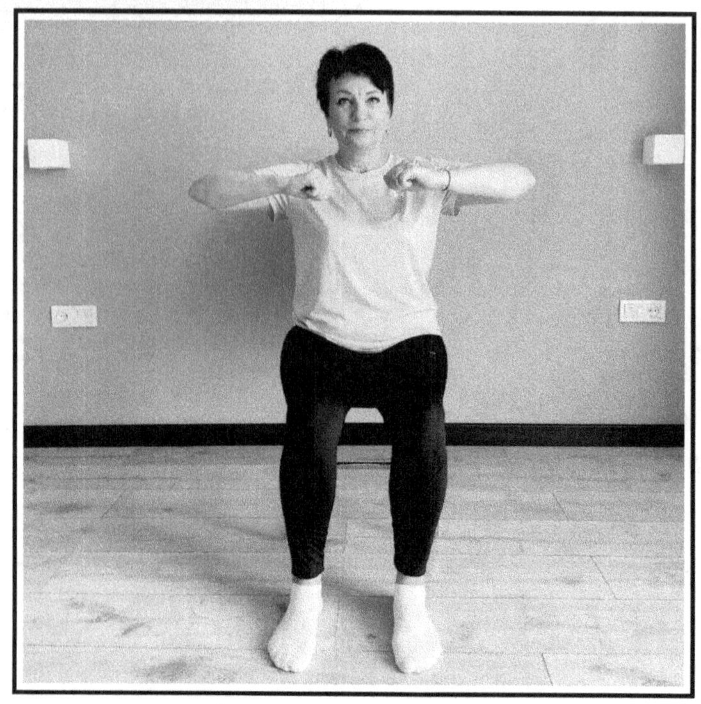
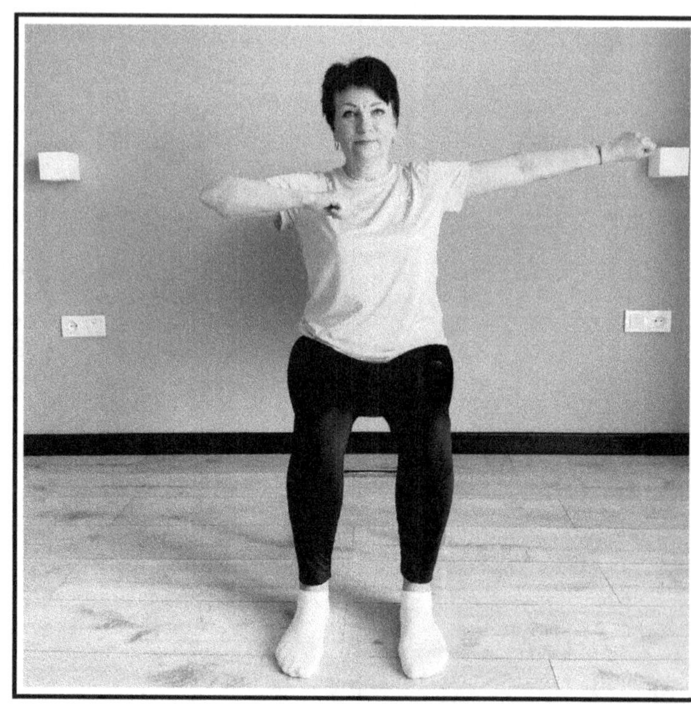

PROCEDURE:

1. Sit tall on the chair
2. Keep your knees bent
3. Put your fists together and bend your elbows to the side
4. From there, open your left arm to the side
5. Bring it back to the starting position
6. Repeat the movement
7. Perform the same exercise with the right arm

SUGGESTED TIPS:

- Don't go too fast
- Don't hold the breath
- Maintain regular breathing while doing this exercise

Exercises for Legs and Hips

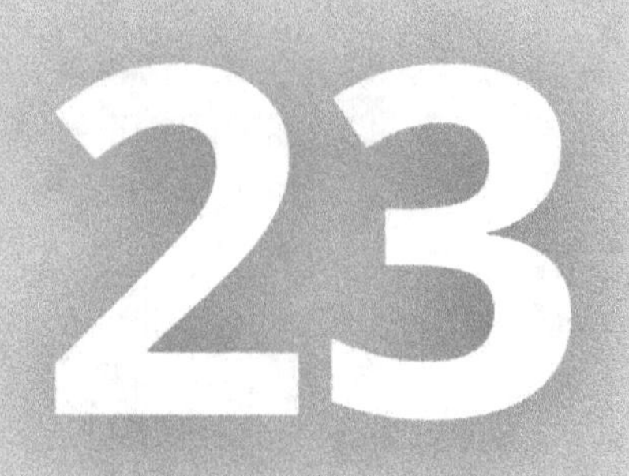

23 Hip Openers

Hip Openers improve your hip mobility. They also activate your glute muscles.

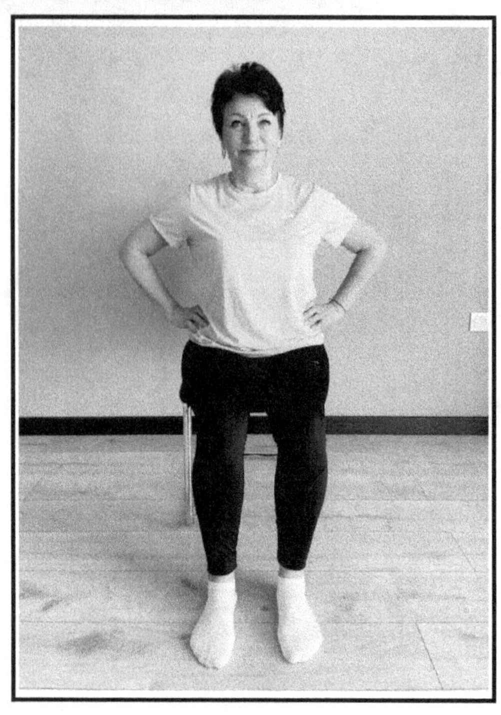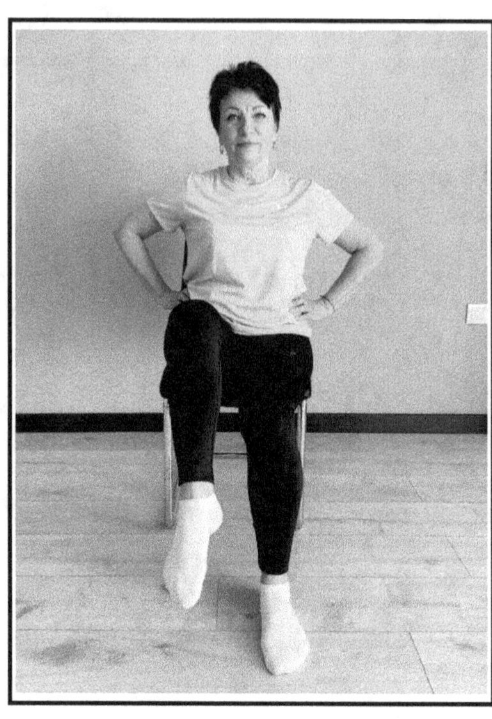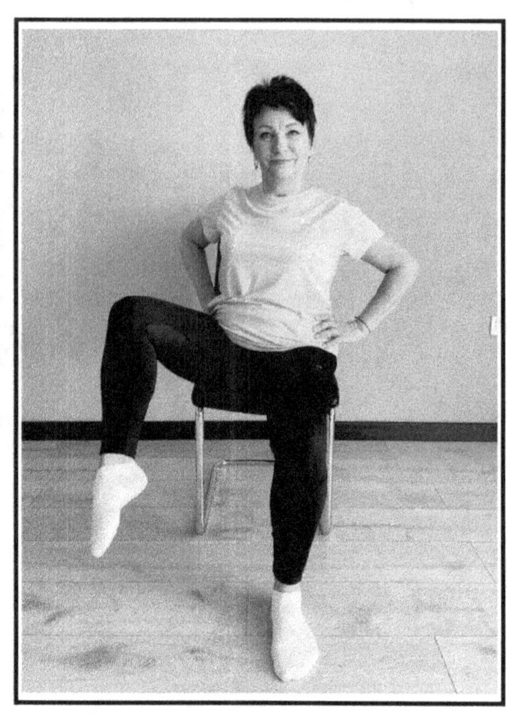

PROCEDURE:

1. Sit tall on the chair
2. Keep your knees bent
3. Keep your hands on your waist
4. Stay in this position; open your leg to the side as far as you can
5. Go back to the previous position and change legs
6. Keep alternating between sides

SUGGESTED TIPS:

- Don't hold the breath
- Don't rush the movement
- Maintain regular breathing throughout this exercise

Knee Extension (Right, Left)

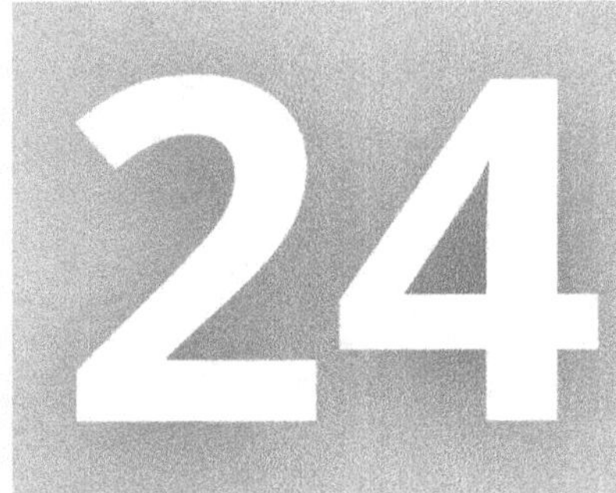

This exercise activates your quadricep muscles. It also strengthens your knee tendons and gives a nice stretch in the hamstring and calf muscles.

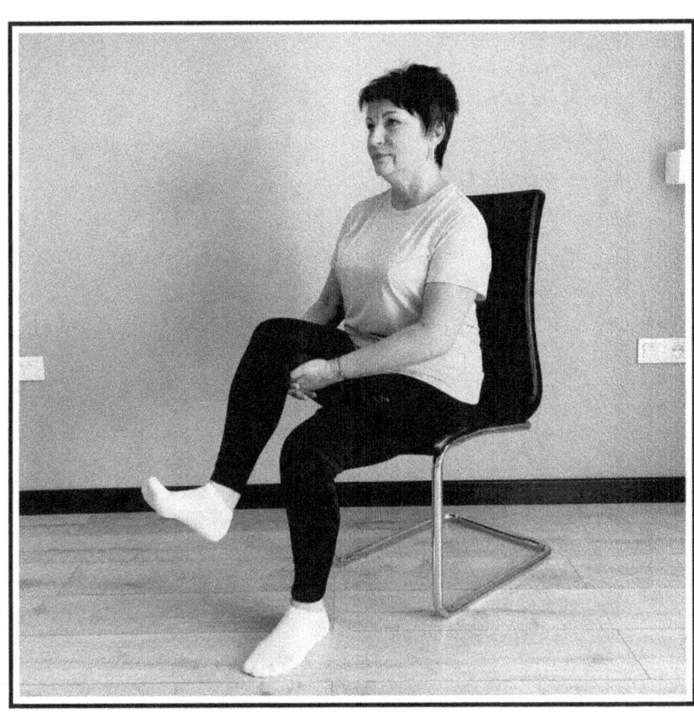 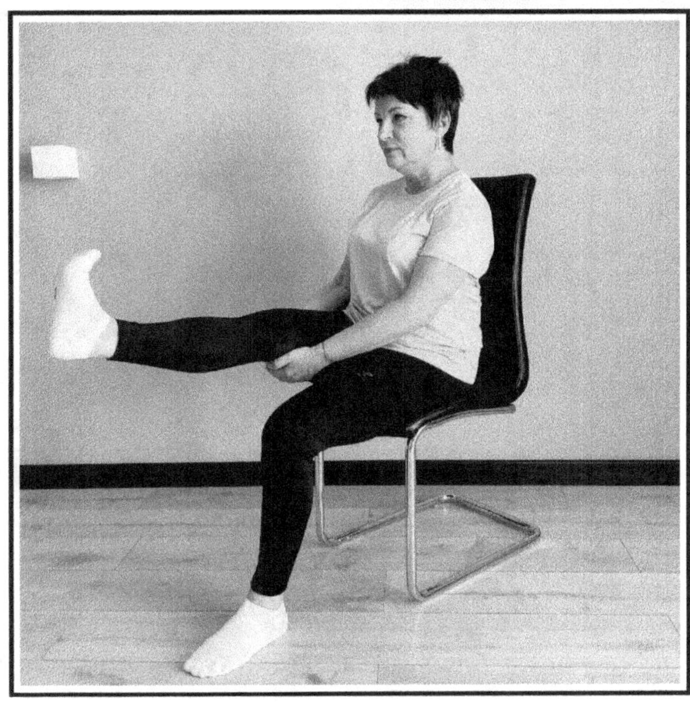

PROCEDURE:

1. Sit tall on the chair with bent knees
2. Grab and lift your right leg with both hands; inhale
3. Extend your right leg forward; exhale
4. Repeat the movement
5. Perform the same exercise with the left leg

SUGGESTED TIPS:

- Don't bend the spine
- Don't hold the breath
- Don't extend your leg too quickly
- Use proper form and be in control when performing this exercise

25 Alternating Seated Leg Extension

This is a fantastic exercise that activates your quadricep muscles and tendons.

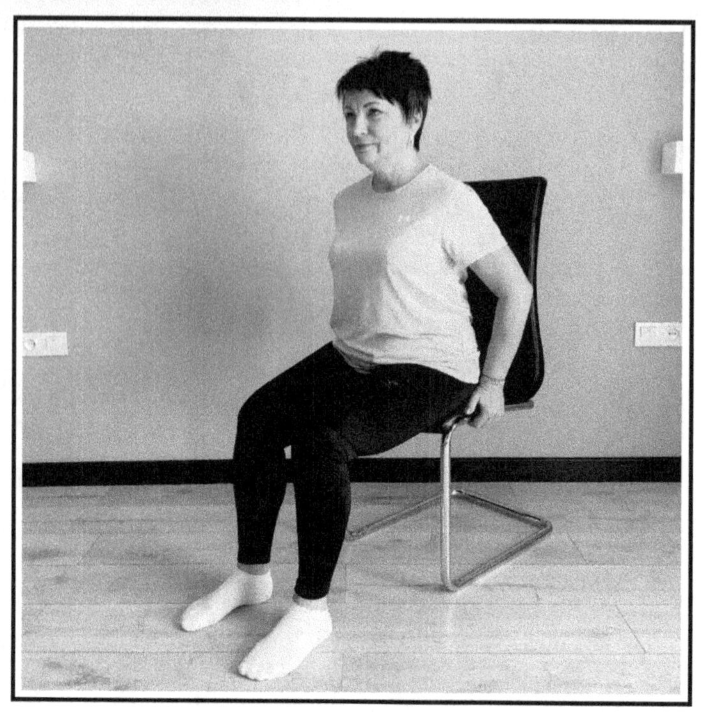

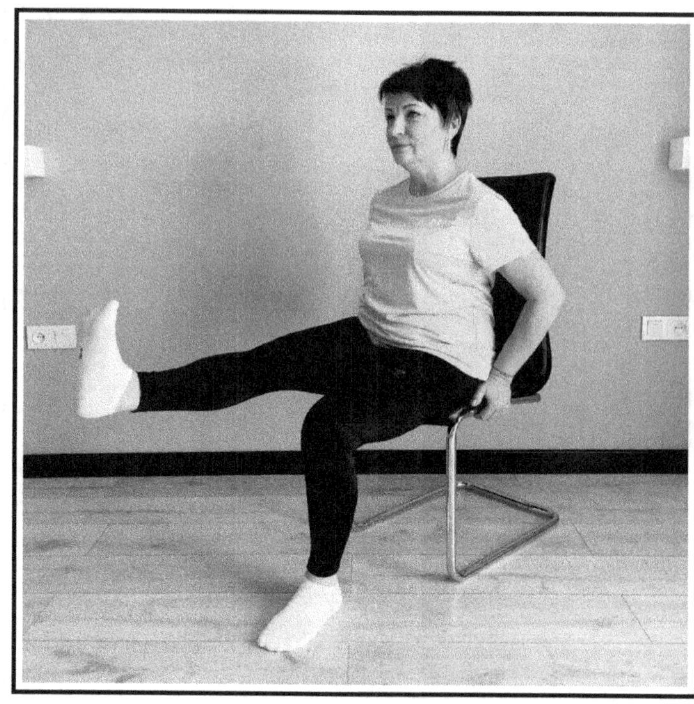

PROCEDURE:

1. Sit tall on the chair with your lower back touching the chair
2. Hold the sides of the chair with your hands; inhale
3. Lift and extend one leg forward; slowly exhale
4. Alternate between legs

SUGGESTED TIPS:

- Don't hold the breath
- Don't go too fast
- Make sure to have maximum control throughout this exercise; go nice and slow

Double Leg Extension

This is a fantastic exercise that activates your quadricep muscles and tendons.

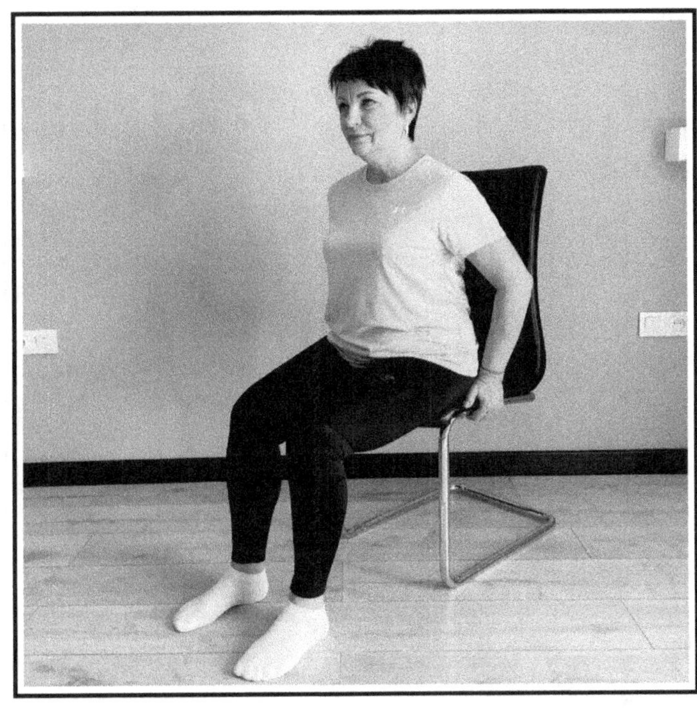 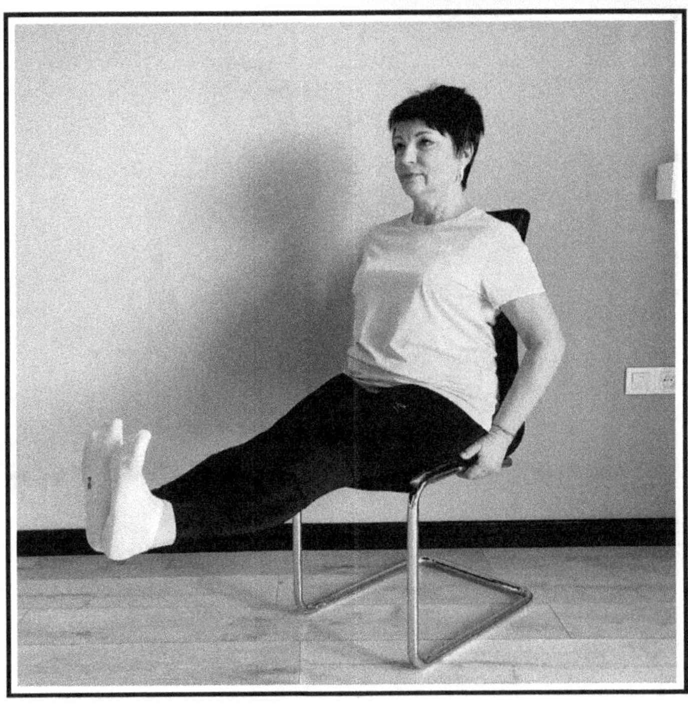

PROCEDURE:

1. Sit tall on the chair with your lower back touching the chair
2. Hold the chair to the sides with your hands; inhale
3. Simultaneously, lift and extend both legs, then exhale
4. Repeat the movement

SUGGESTED TIPS:

- Don't move your back from the chair
- Don't hold the breath
- Don't go too fast
- Make sure to have maximum control throughout this exercise; go nice and slow

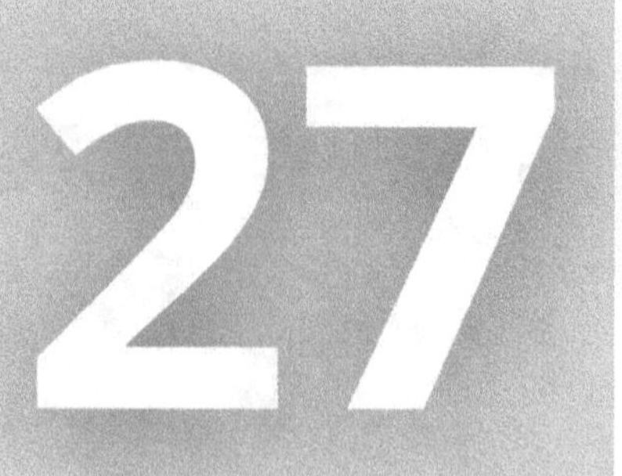

27 Foot Flexion + Extension
(Right, Left)

This exercise works your ankle mobility. It also activates and stretches your calf muscles.

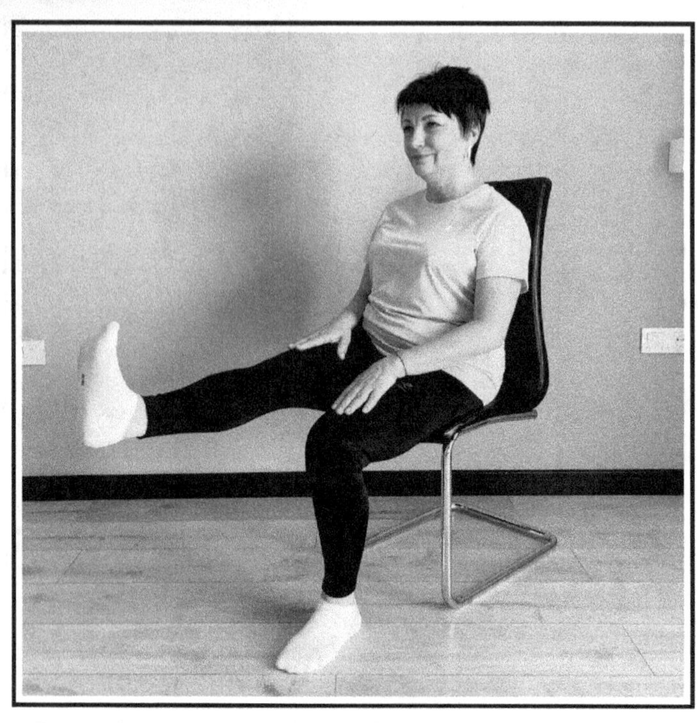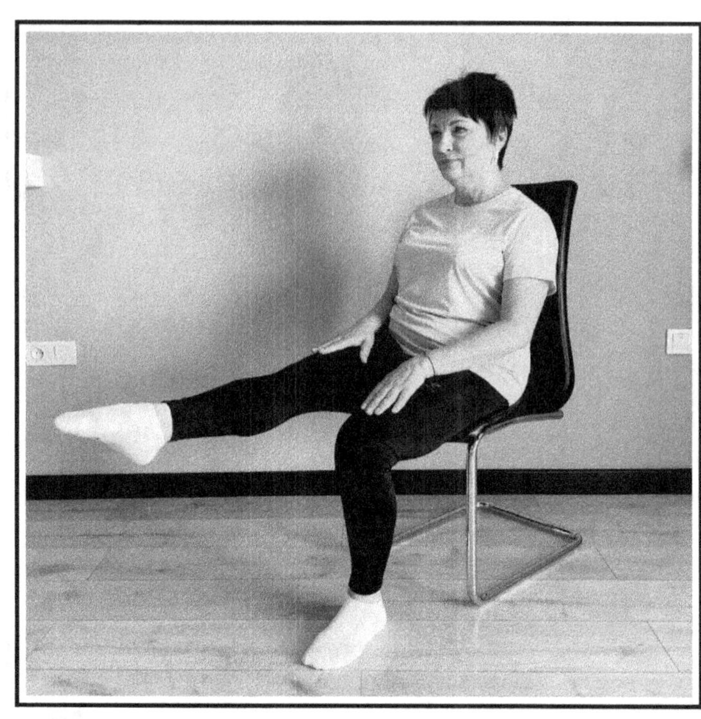

PROCEDURE:

1. Sit tall on the chair; keep your knees bent
2. Lift and extend your right leg
3. Point your right toes up
4. Point your right toes down
5. Repeat the movement
6. Perform the same exercise with the left leg

SUGGESTED TIPS:

- Don't do the movement too fast
- Don't hold the breath
- Don't arch the spine
- Don't rush while doing this exercise
- Follow the tempo of this exercise (i.e., medium – not too fast or too slow)

Heel Raises to Toes Raises

This is a great exercise that works your calf muscles. It also strengthens your ankles.

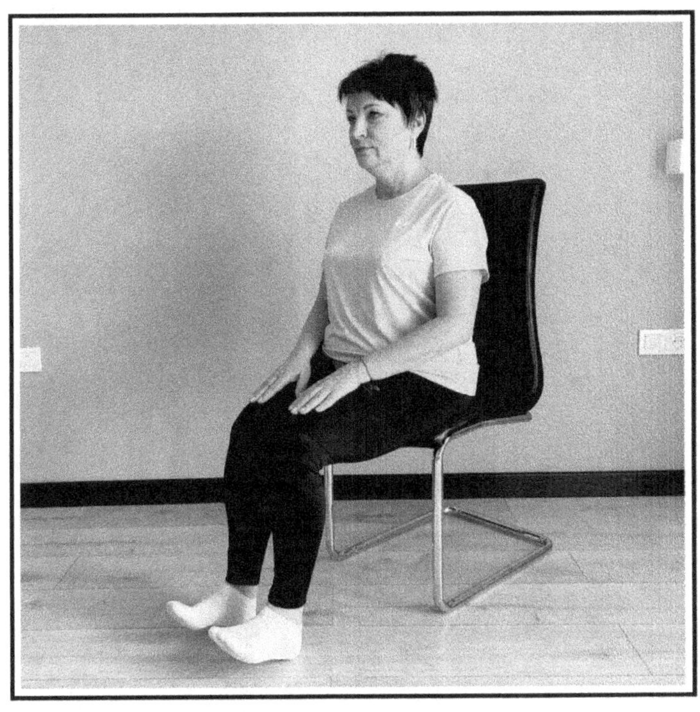 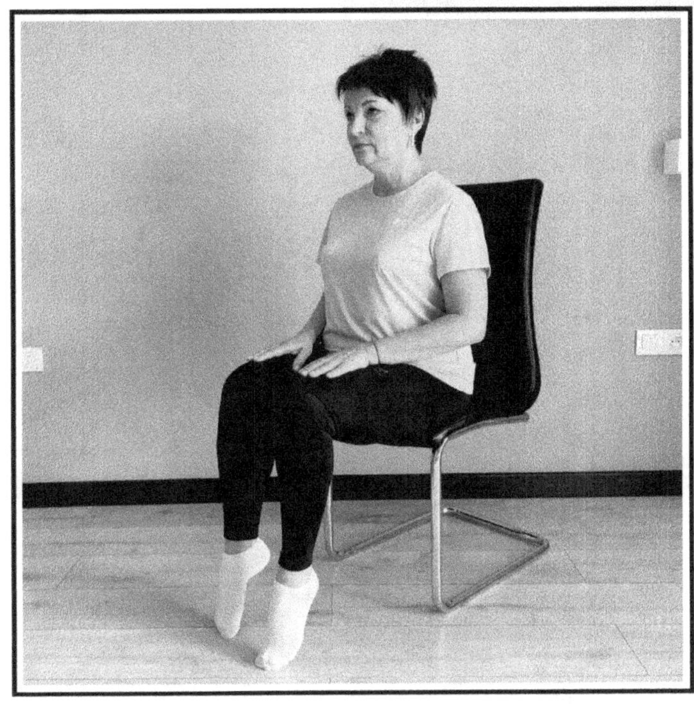

PROCEDURE:

1. Sit tall on the chair with bent knees
2. Lift your heels up
3. Bring your heels down and lift your toes up
4. Repeat the exercise

SUGGESTED TIPS:

- Don't go too fast
- Don't hold the breath
- Don't arch the back
- Don't rush performing this exercise
- Perform the exercise slowly with full control while maintaining regular breathing

Exercises for Back

Bodyweight Rows

Bodyweight Rows strengthen your upper back muscles.

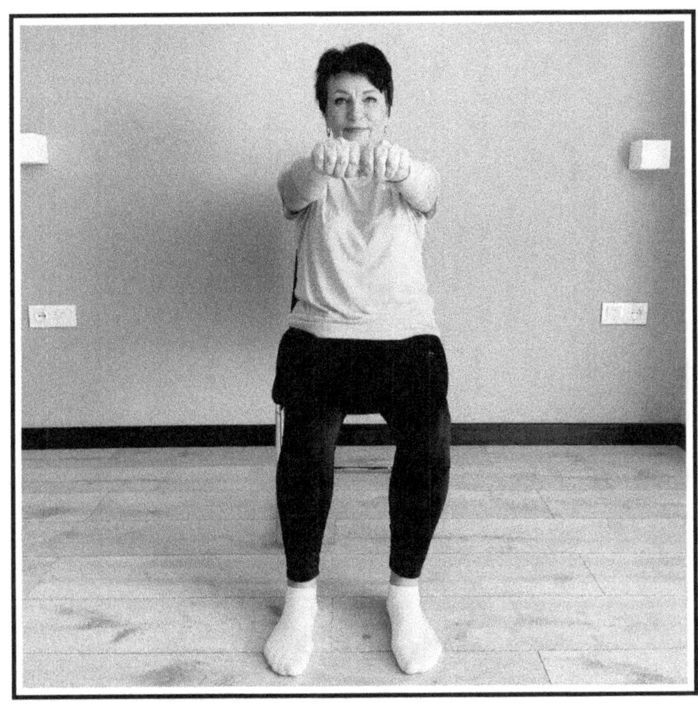 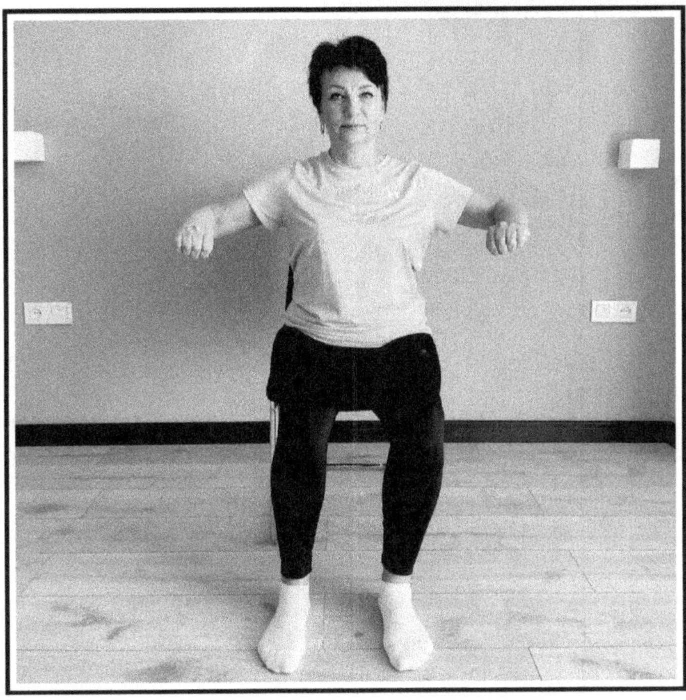

PROCEDURE:

1. Sit tall on the chair
2. Keep your knees bent
3. Extend your arms out forward as much as you can; inhale
4. Exhale, and pull your hands backward while squeezing your shoulder blades
5. Repeat the exercise

SUGGESTED TIPS:

- Don't arch the spine
- Don't go too fast
- Don't hold the breath
- Bring your elbows to a 45-degree angle to activate more of your mid-back muscles

Spinal Twist (Right, Left)

Spinal twist is a fantastic exercise that makes your thoracic part of the spine more mobile. It also improves your lower back mobility.

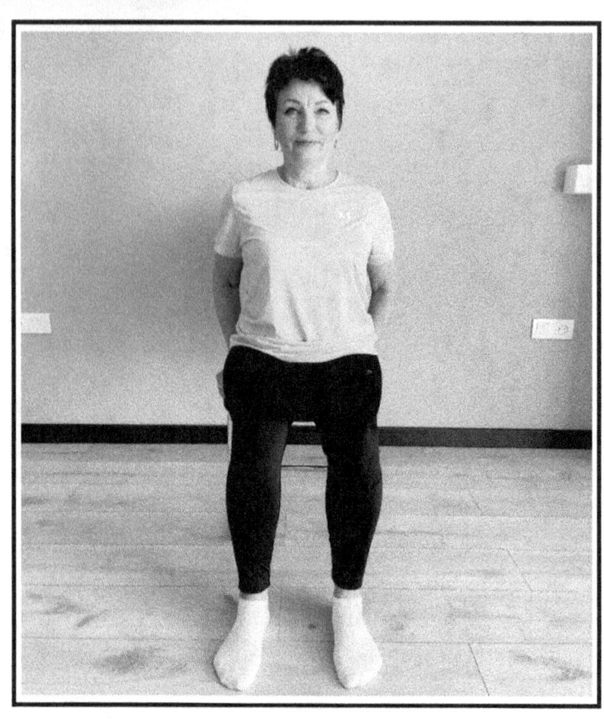 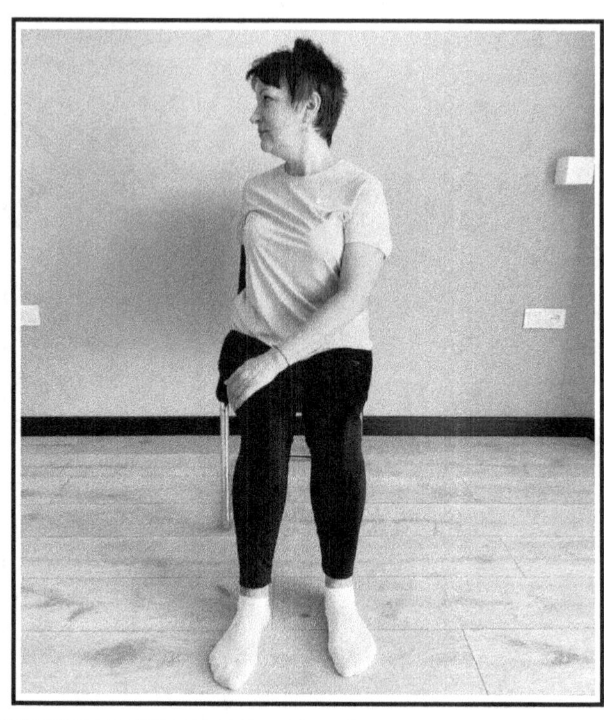

PROCEDURE:

1. Sit tall on the chair; keep your knees bent
2. Put your hands on your knees
3. Put the right hand on the backside of the chair and twist your body to the right side
4. Place your left hand on the outward part of your right knee, and push off of it
5. Hold this stretch
6. Perform the same exercise on the other side

SUGGESTED TIPS:

- Don't rush the movement
- Don't hold the breath
- Make sure to take a deep breath and exhale once you start twisting your body to the side

PAGE 50

Side Bends

This is a fantastic exercise that stretches the sides of your abdominals and your back.

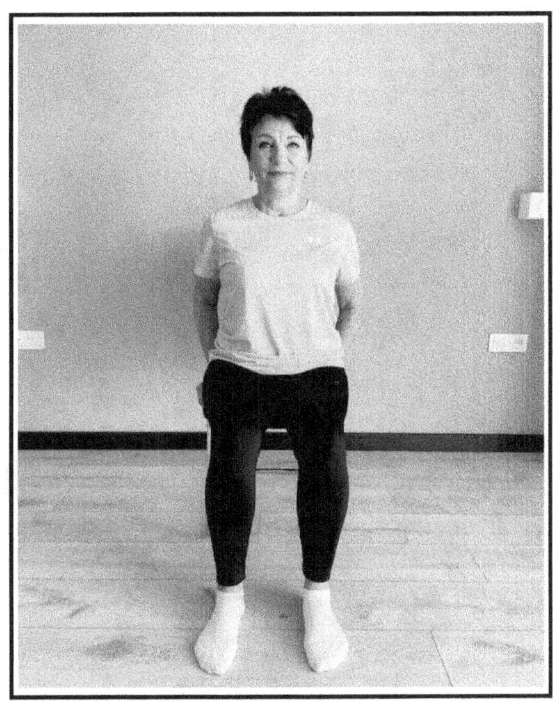 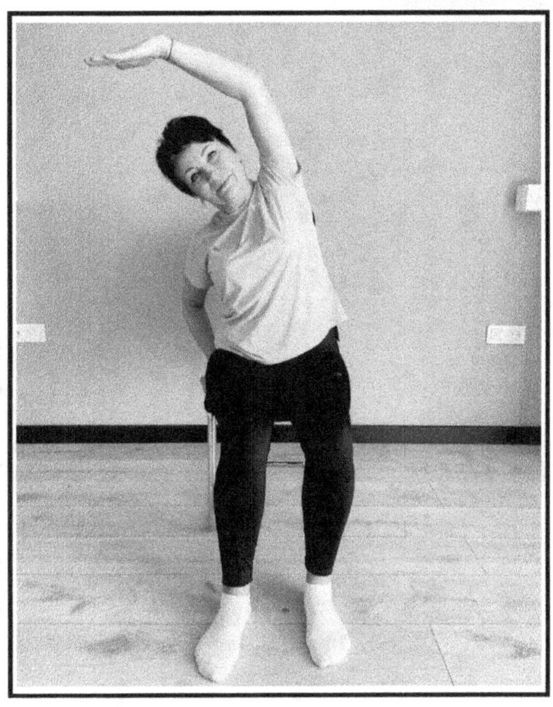

1. Sit tall on the chair
2. Keep your knees bent
3. Keep left arm extended next to your side; inhale
4. Bend your body to the left side and swing your right arm across the head; exhale
5. Go back to the neutral position
6. Alternate between sides

- Don't go too fast
- Don't hold the breath
- Take your time and do the exercise with maximum control

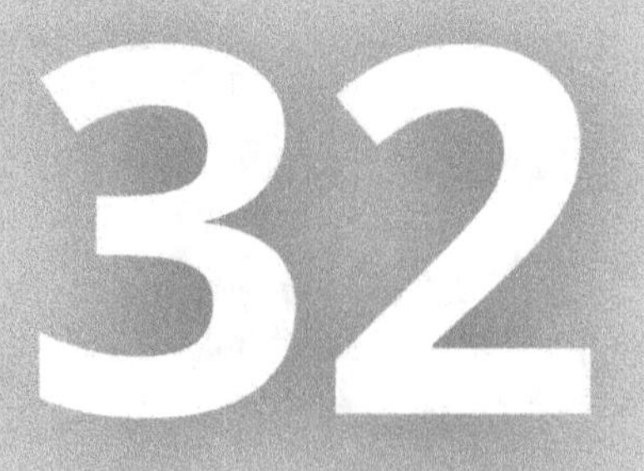 # Side Reach

This is a good exercise that stretches the side of your body.

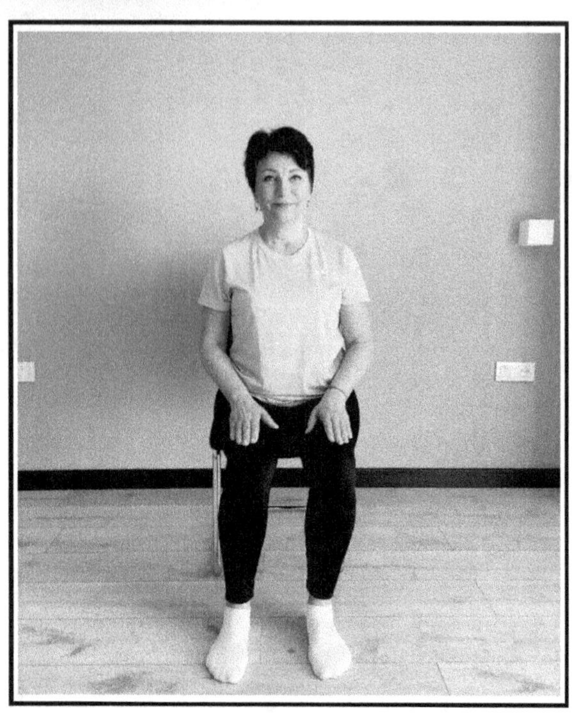 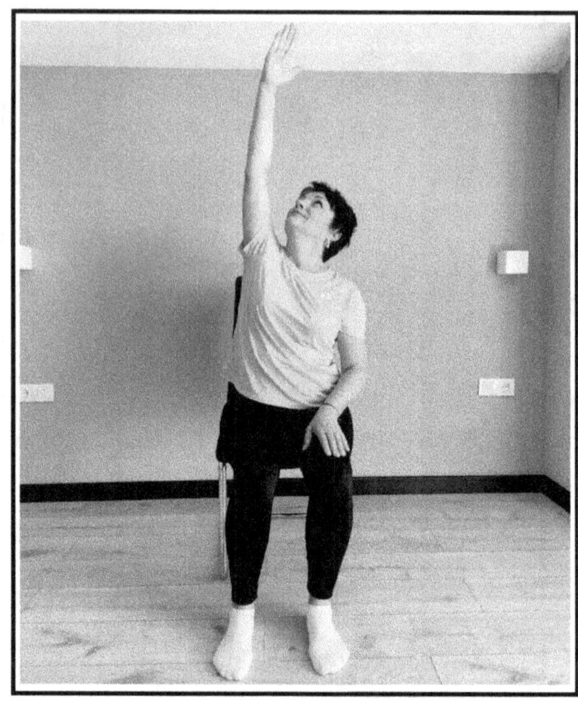

PROCEDURE:

1. Sit tall on the chair
2. Keep your knees bent
3. Lift your left arm, and pretend you are reaching something high up
4. Gently bend your body to the right side
5. Alternate between sides

SUGGESTED TIPS:

- Don't hold the breath
- Don't bend the spine
- Maintain regular breathing while doing this exercise

Thoracic Rotations

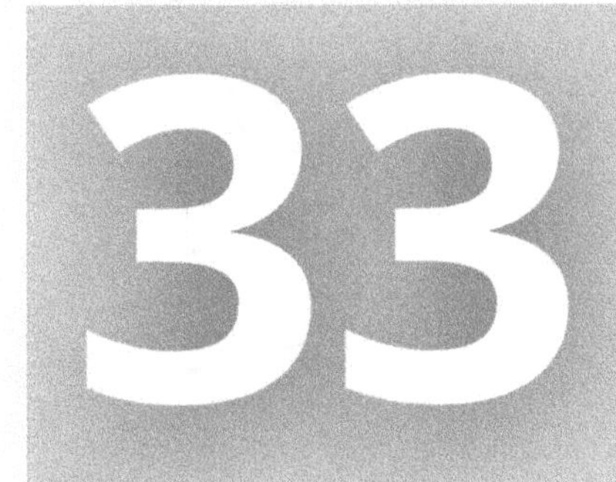

This is a phenomenal exercise to relieve the tightness in your upper and mid-back.

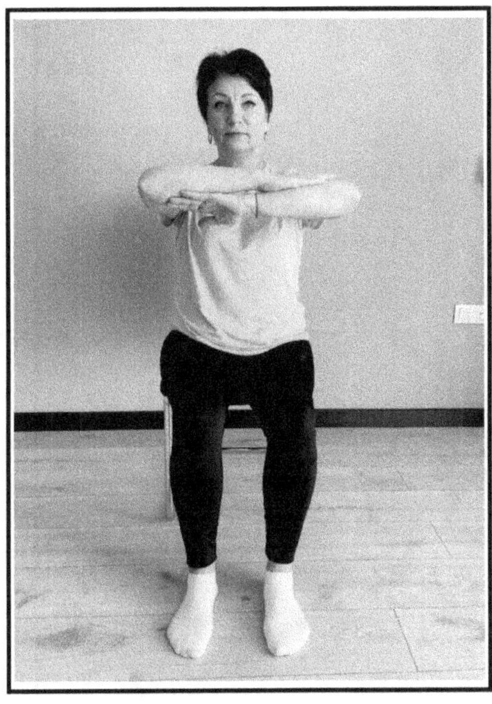 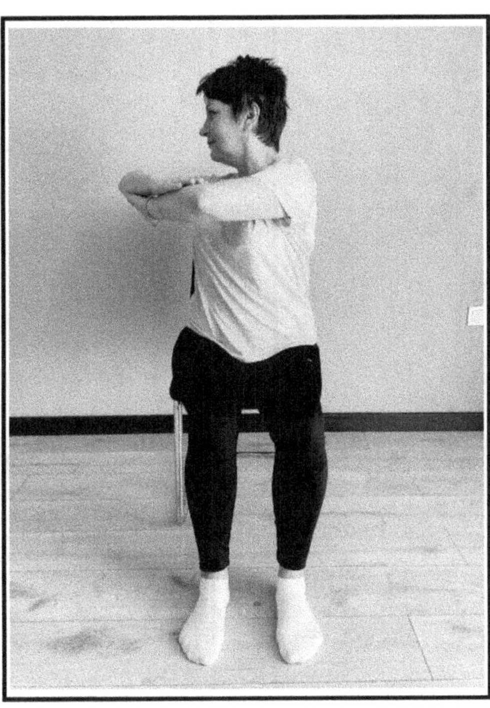 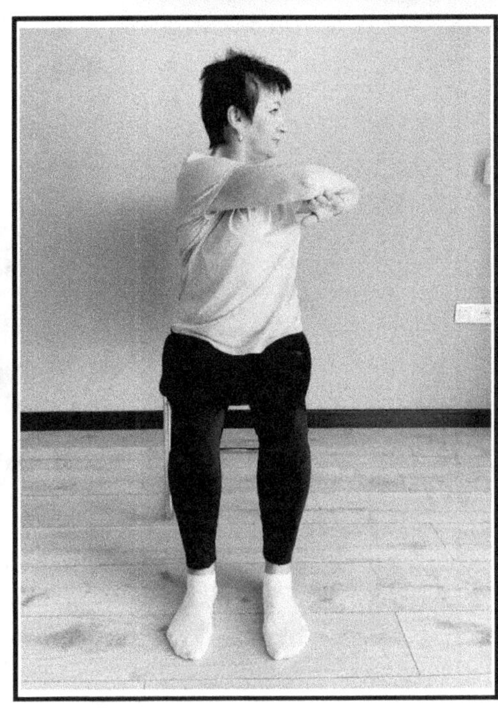

PROCEDURE:

1. Sit tall on the chair
2. Keep your knees bent
3. Put your elbows on top of each other
4. Inhale and tighten your core
5. Exhale and twist your body to one side, making sure your head follows your body movement
6. Alternate between sides

SUGGESTED TIPS:

- Don't hold the breath
- Follow the movement with your head
- Don't rush the movement in this exercise
- Start slow with full control

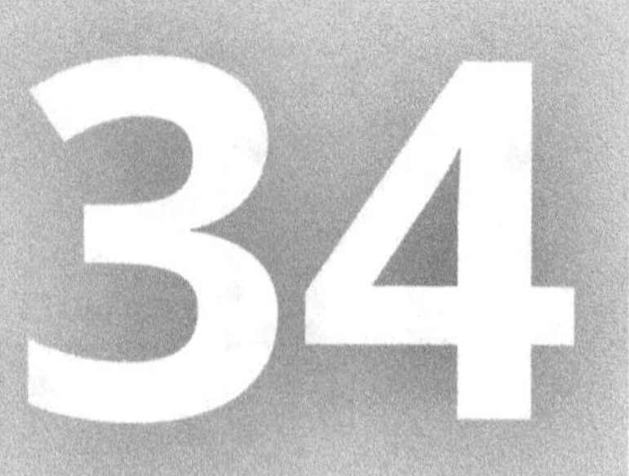

34 Thoracic Mobility

This exercise will improve your upper back mobility and reset your posture.

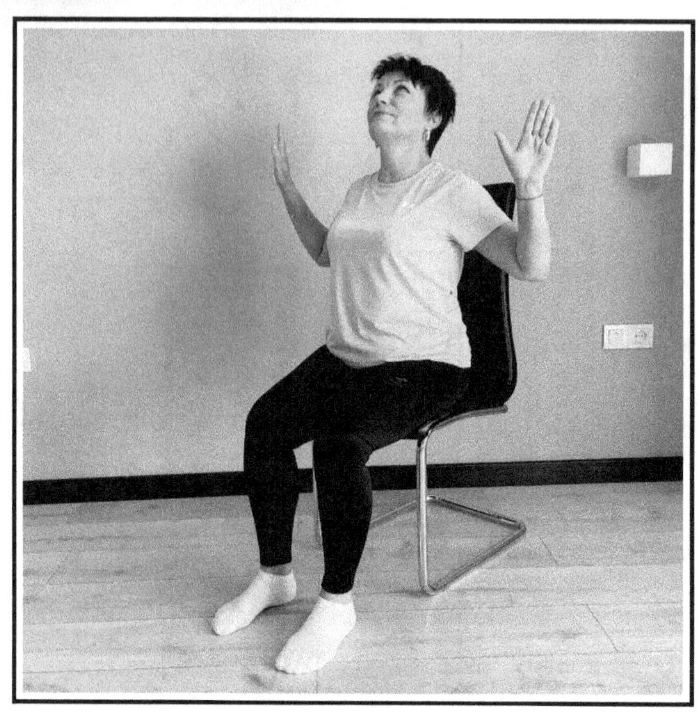
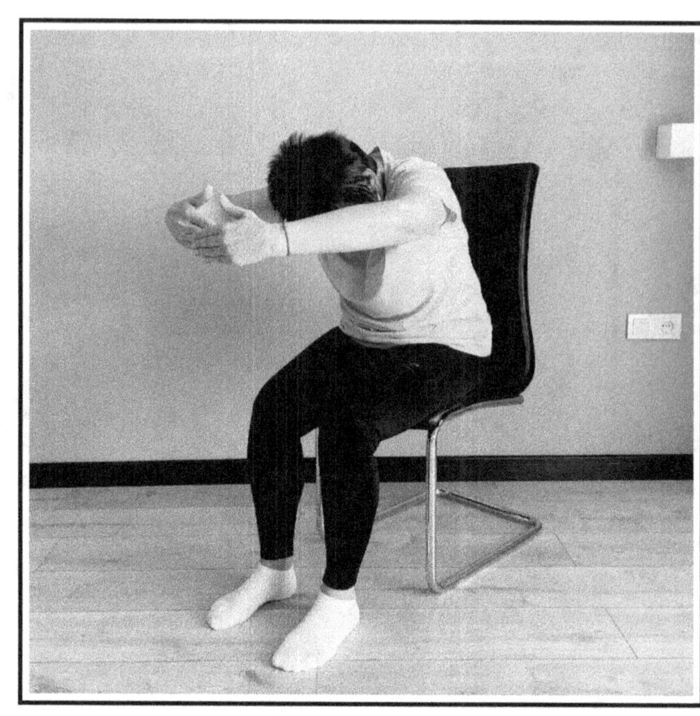

PROCEDURE:

1. Sit tall on the chair; keep your knees bent
2. Extend your arms out forward and rotate your hands so that the backside of your palms is touching
3. Gently round your upper back and bend the neck
4. From there, open your chest up, and bring your arms up behind you
5. Repeat the movement

SUGGESTED TIPS:

- Don't rush the movement
- Don't hold the breath
- Follow the movement with your head
- Inhale while you are keeping your neck bent
- Exhale as you start opening up your chest

PAGE 54

Chair Sun Salutation

This exercise mobilizes your upper and lower back. It's great to do after sitting down for an extended time.

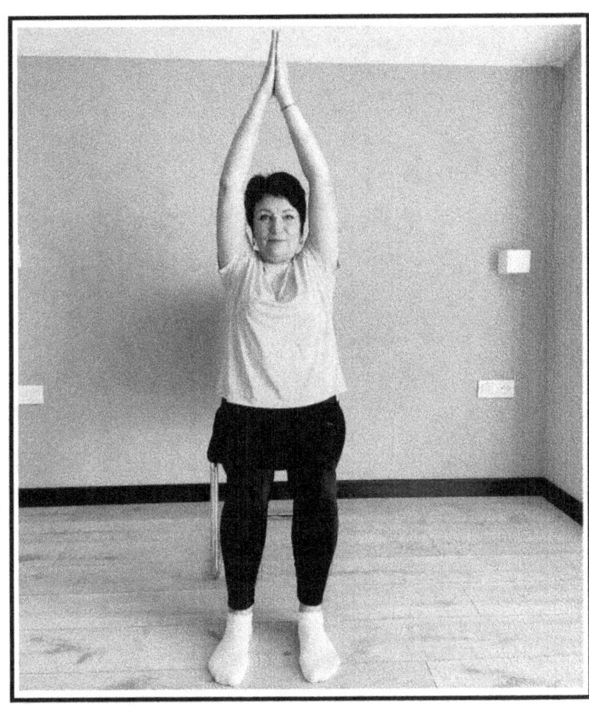
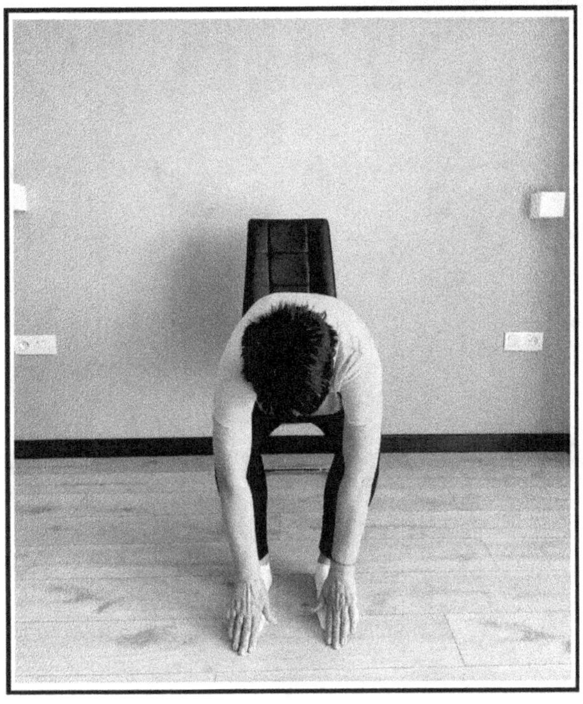

PROCEDURE:

1. Sit on the chair with your posture tall
2. Lift your arms up and above your head
3. Bend your body forward and touch your feet with your hands
4. Extend your neck and upper back, and go to the starting position
5. Repeat the movement

SUGGESTED TIPS:

- Don't rush the movement
- Try breathing from the stomach throughout this exercise

36 Back Folds

This is a good exercise that mobilizes your lower and upper back.

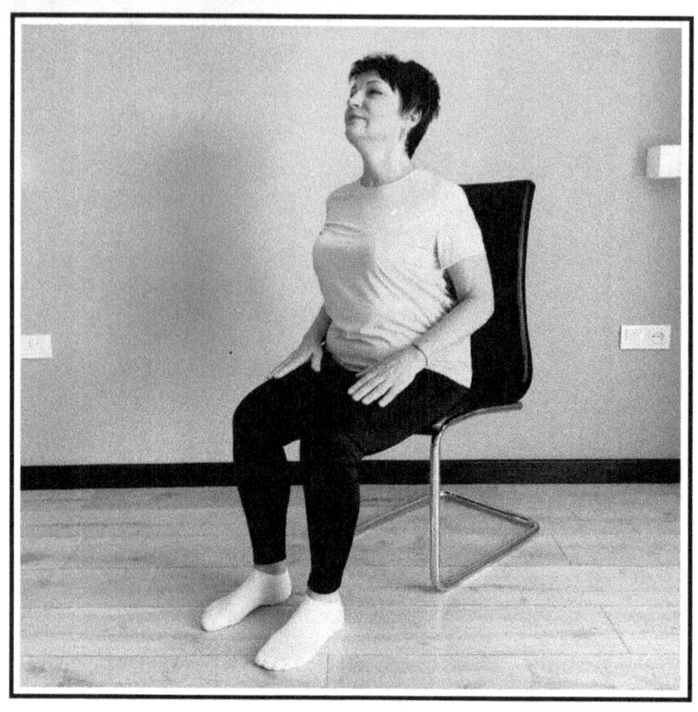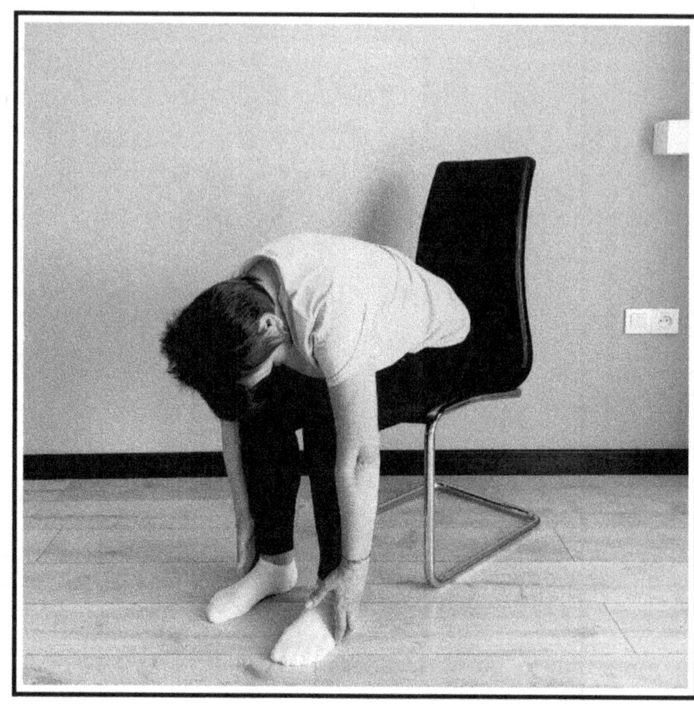

PROCEDURE:

1. Sit tall on the chair
2. Keep your knees bent and spread them apart
3. Put your hands on your knees
4. From this position, push your back backward
5. Fold your body in between your legs (let your hands slide over your shins and make sure your head follows the movement)
6. Slowly rise up to the starting position and roll your shoulders backward; repeat the movement

SUGGESTED TIPS:

- Follow the movement with your head
- Don't go too fast; don't hold the breath
- Inhale at the beginning of the movement
- Slowly exhale as you start folding your body forward
- Inhale again from the bottom position
- Exhale as you start going up

Full Body Exercises

37 Dynamic Hamstring Stretch

As the name says, this exercise dynamically stretches your hamstrings and calves.

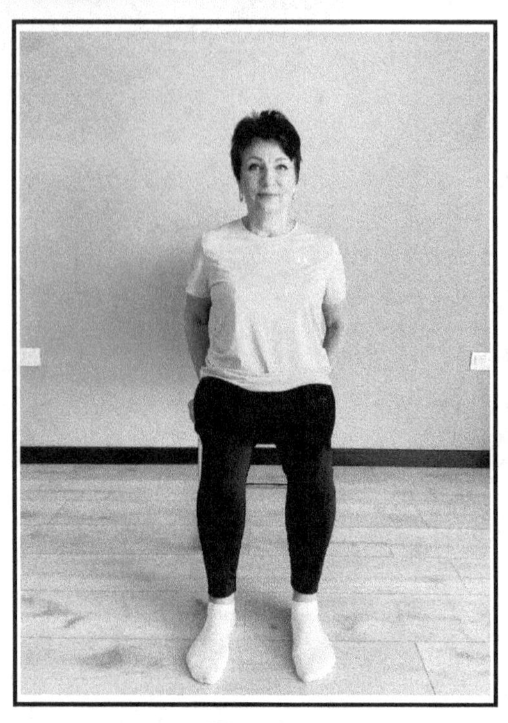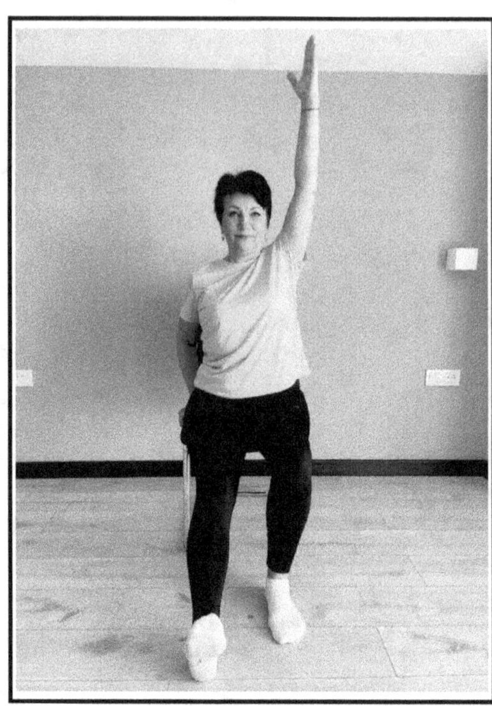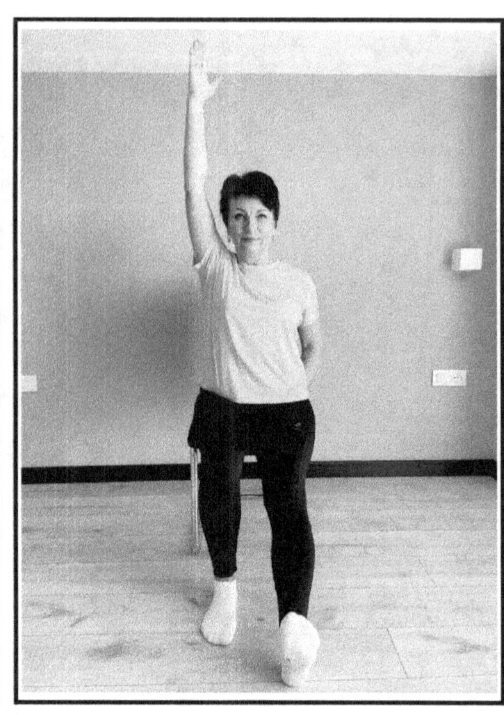

PROCEDURE:

1. Sit tall on the chair
2. Keep your knees bent; inhale
3. Take your left arm and bring it all the way up
4. Extend your right leg forward; keep your toes pointing up and your heel on the ground
5. Exhale; bring your arm down
6. Alternate between sides

SUGGESTED TIPS:

- Don't bend the knee; don't arch the lower back
- Point the toes up
- Don't hold the breath
- Inhale before you lift your arm up
- Exhale as you start bringing the arm down

Seated Punches

Seated Punches work your coordination. This exercise also works your arm muscles and hip flexors.

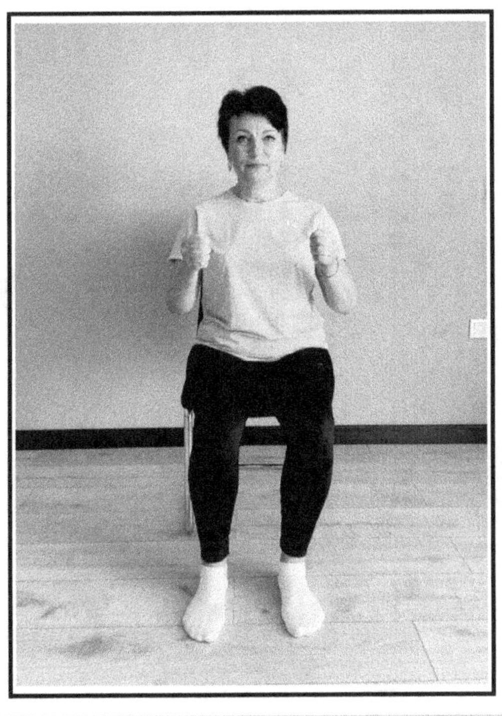 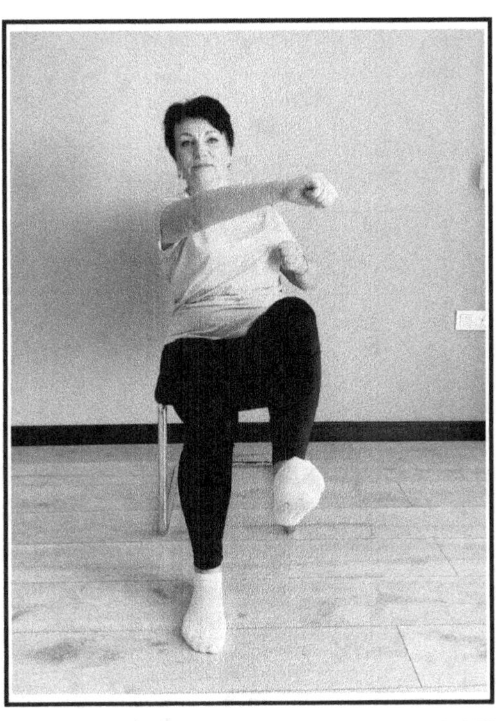 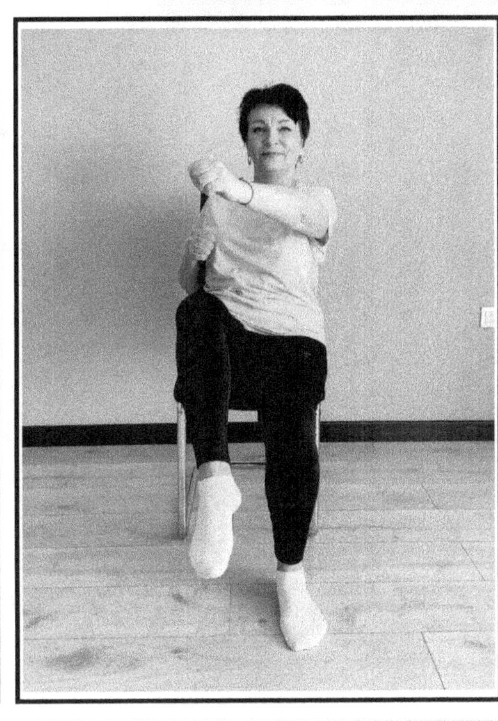

PROCEDURE:

1. Sit tall on the chair; keep your knees bent
2. Keep your hands next to your body
3. Simultaneously, lift your left knee and punch to your left side with your right hand
4. Go back to the starting position and mirror the movement on the other side
5. Alternate between sides

SUGGESTED TIPS:

- Don't go too fast
- Don't hold the breath
- At the beginning of the movement, inhale
- Exhale as you start punching to the side

39 Seated Marching

Seated Marching is a great exercise that works your cardiovascular system. It's also a fantastic way to warm up.

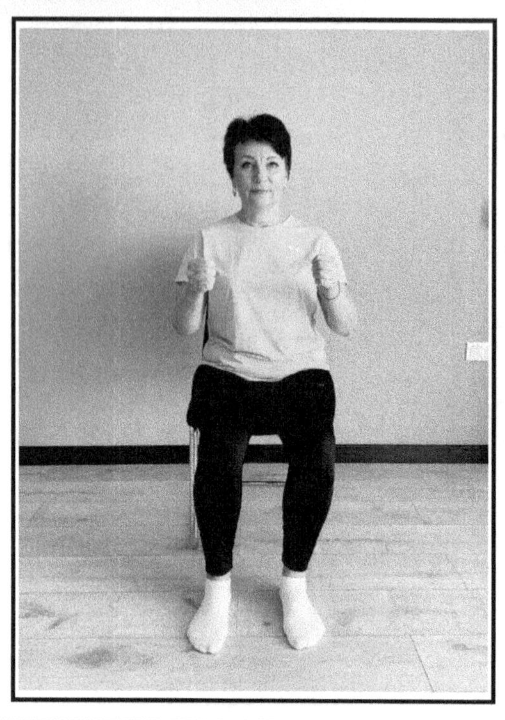 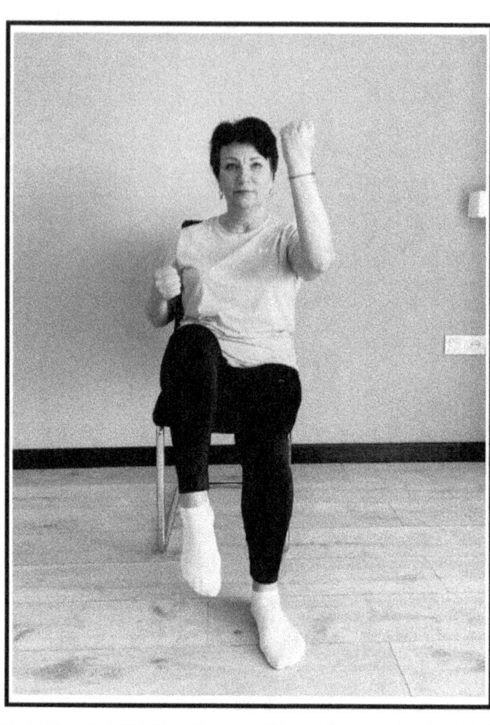 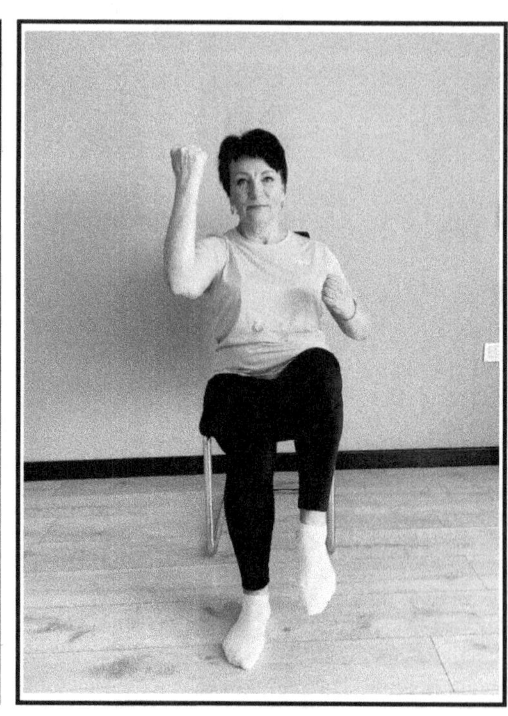

PROCEDURE:

1. Sit tall on the chair
2. Keep your knees bent
3. Keep your hands at your sides
4. Bend your left elbow and punch up
5. Lift your right leg in the knee, while keeping the other leg bent
6. Go back to the previous position
7. Alternate between sides

SUGGESTED TIPS:

- Don't rush the movement
- Don't hold the breath
- Maintain regular breathing while doing this exercise

Arm Pulldowns

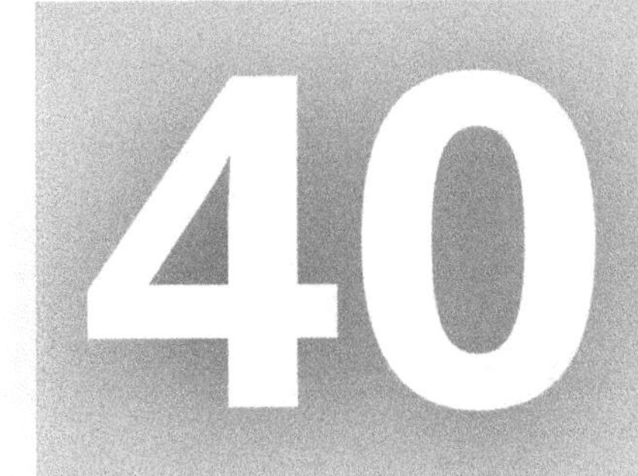

Arm Pulldowns activate your stomach muscles and hip flexors. They also activate your back muscles.

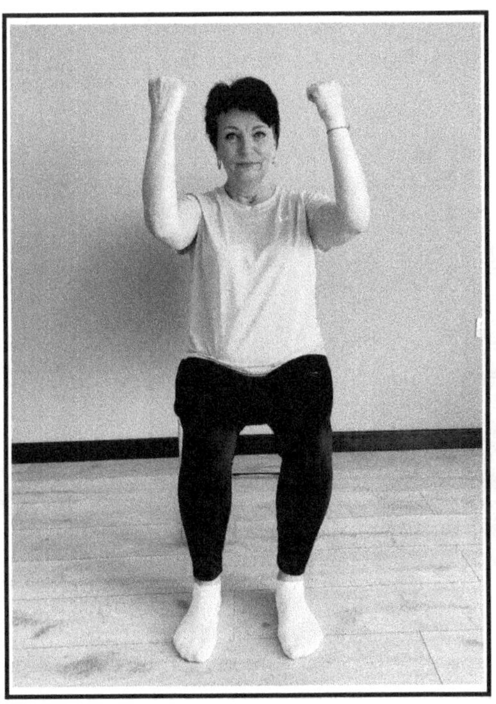 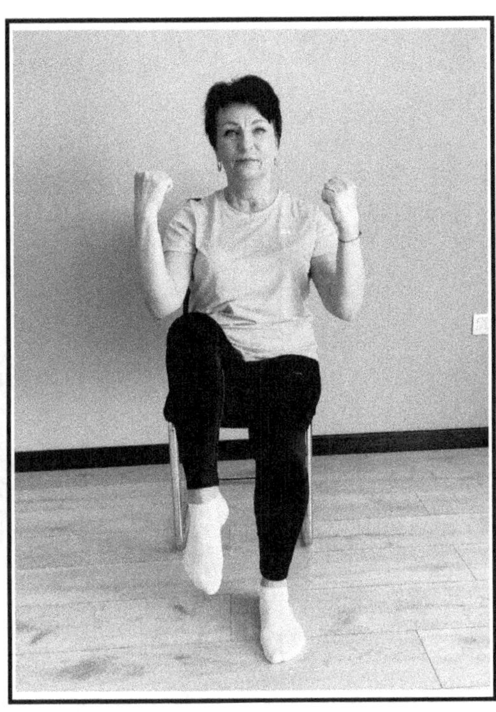 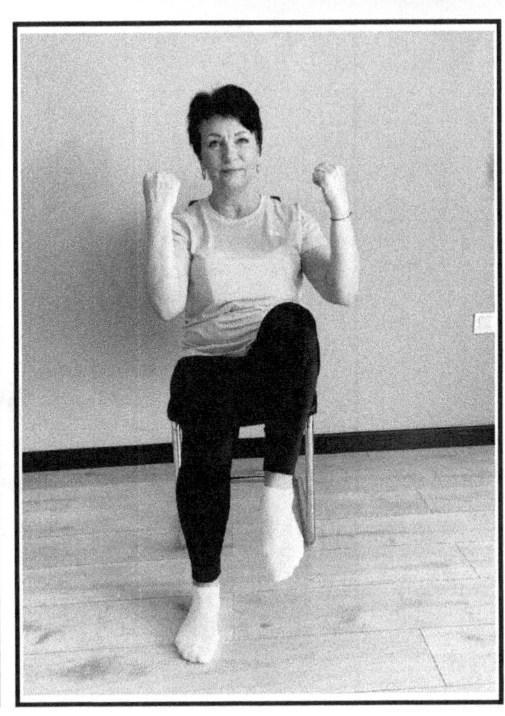

PROCEDURE:

1. Sit tall on the chair
2. Keep your knees bent
3. Lift your elbows up
4. Bring your elbows down while lifting one of your knees up
5. Go to the previous position
6. Alternate between legs

SUGGESTED TIPS:

- Don't hold the breath
- Don't rush the movement
- Inhale, then bring your elbows down
- When you start lifting one knee up, exhale

Around the World

This exercise warms up your upper body. It is a great choice for a warm-up exercise.

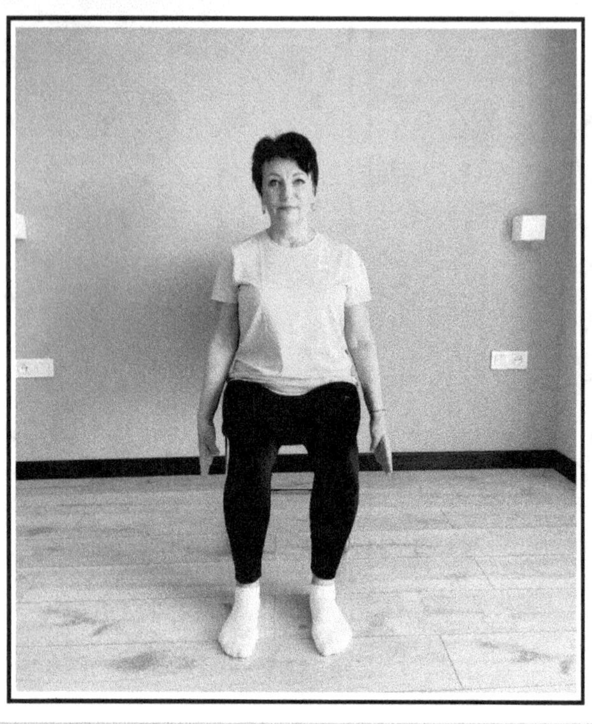
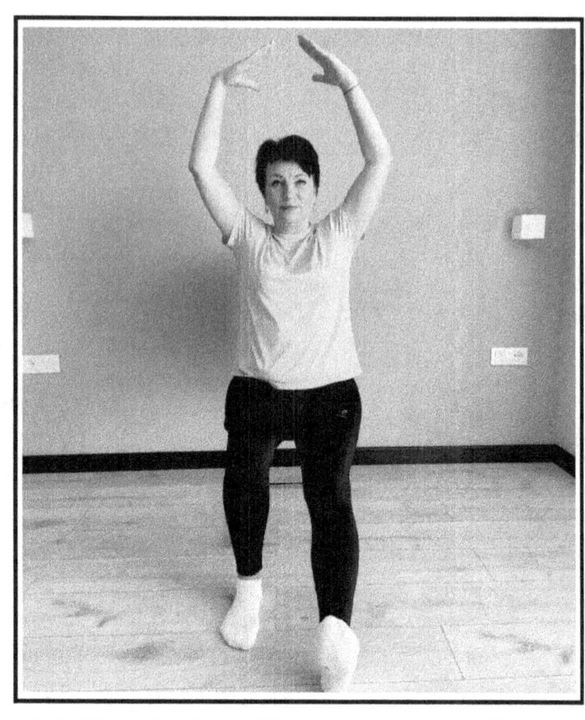

PROCEDURE:

1. Sit tall on the chair
2. Keep your knees bent
3. Keep your arms next to your body with palms facing forward
4. Raise your arms to the side and above your head
5. As you are doing so, step forward with one foot
6. Bring hands and the leg back
7. Repeat alternating between legs

SUGGESTED TIPS:

- Don't rush the movement
- Don't hold the breath
- While doing this exercise, maintain regular breathing

PAGE 62

Marching Arm Pumps

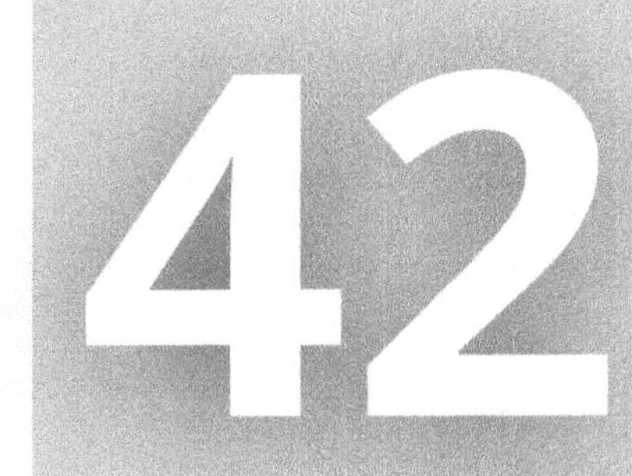

This exercise is a fun, dynamic way to warm up your lower and upper body.

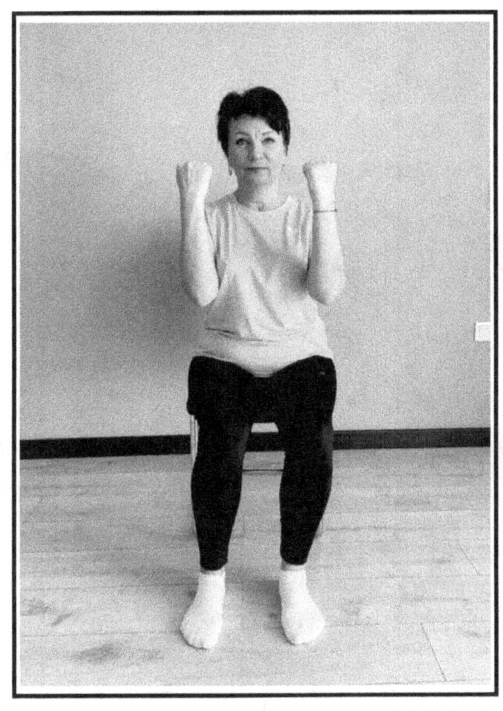 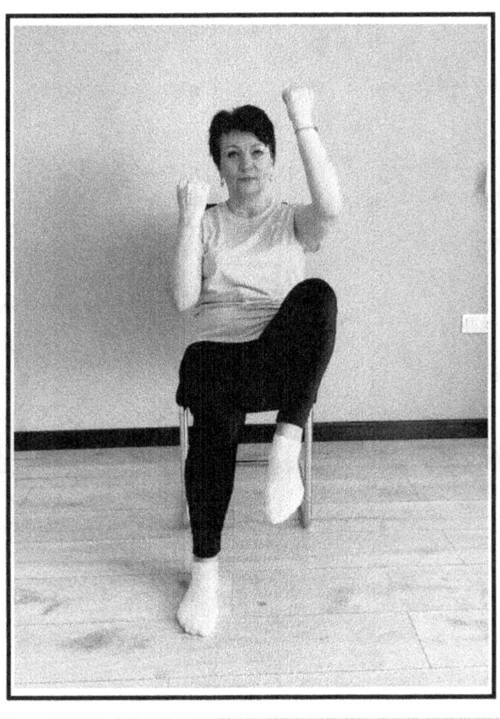 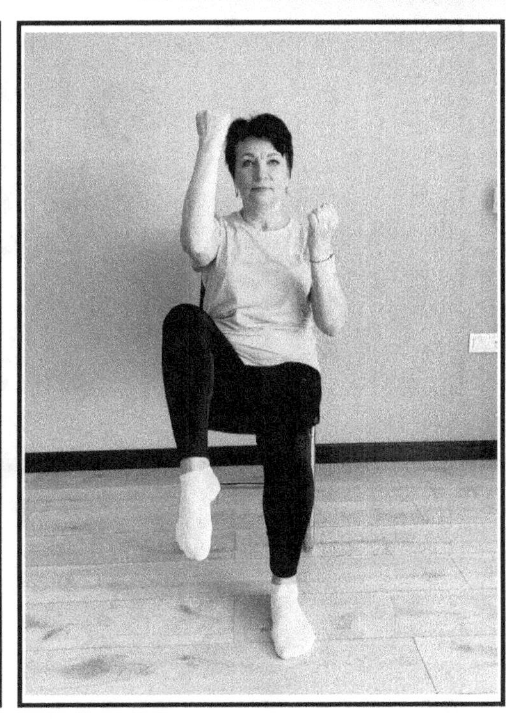

PROCEDURE:

1. Sit tall on the chair
2. Keep your knees bent
3. Simultaneously, lift your left knee, make a fist, and punch up with your left hand
4. Bring the left knee and arm down; do the same movement with your right knee and right arm
5. Alternate between arms and legs

SUGGESTED TIPS:

- Don't rush the movement
- Don't hold the breath
- At the beginning of the movement, inhale
- Exhale as you start punching up

Knee Claps

Knee Claps work your hip flexor muscles and your shoulders.

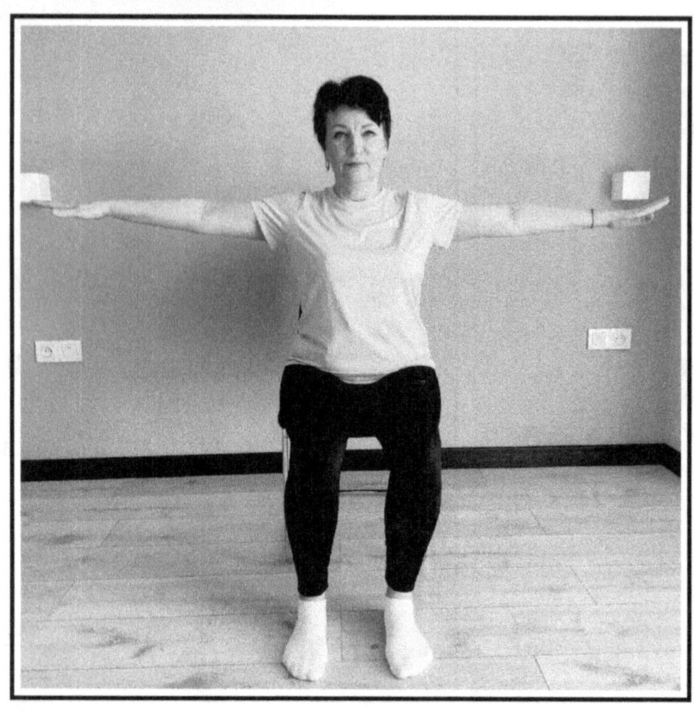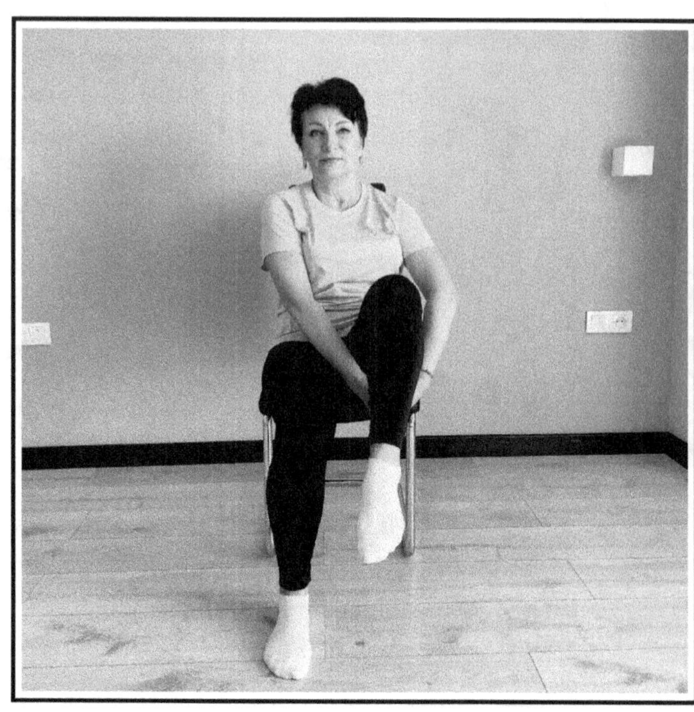

PROCEDURE:

1. Sit tall on the chair
2. Keep your knees bent
3. Lift your arms to the side
4. Lift your left knee up
5. Clap your hands under your left knee
6. Bring the left knee down; repeat the movement with the right knee
7. Alternate between legs

SUGGESTED TIPS:

- Don't hold the breath
- Don't do the movement too slowly unless you experience knee problems
- Maintain regular breathing while doing this exercise

PAGE 64

Elbow to Knee

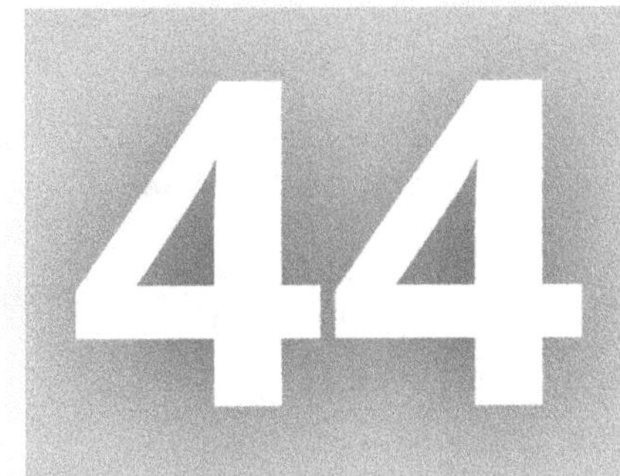

This is a fantastic exercise that works your side abdominal muscles and mobilizes your lower back.

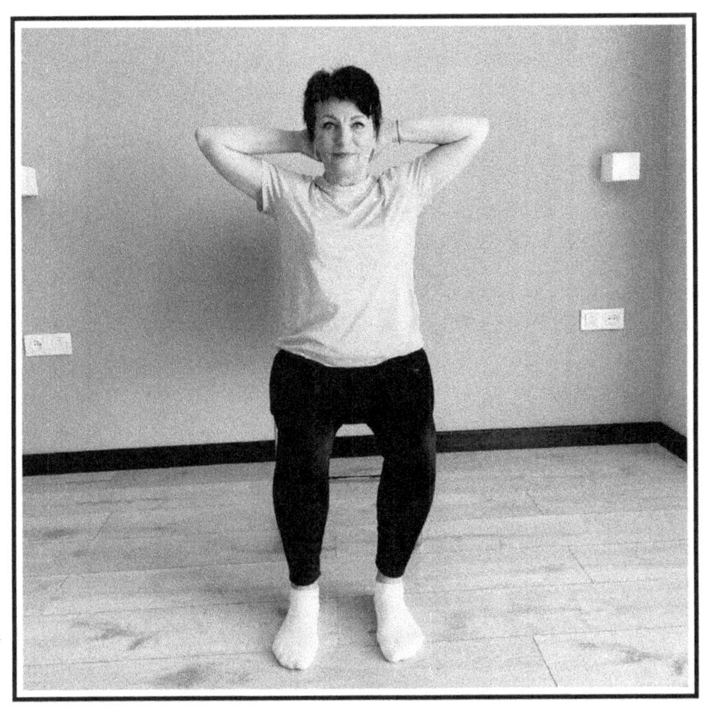

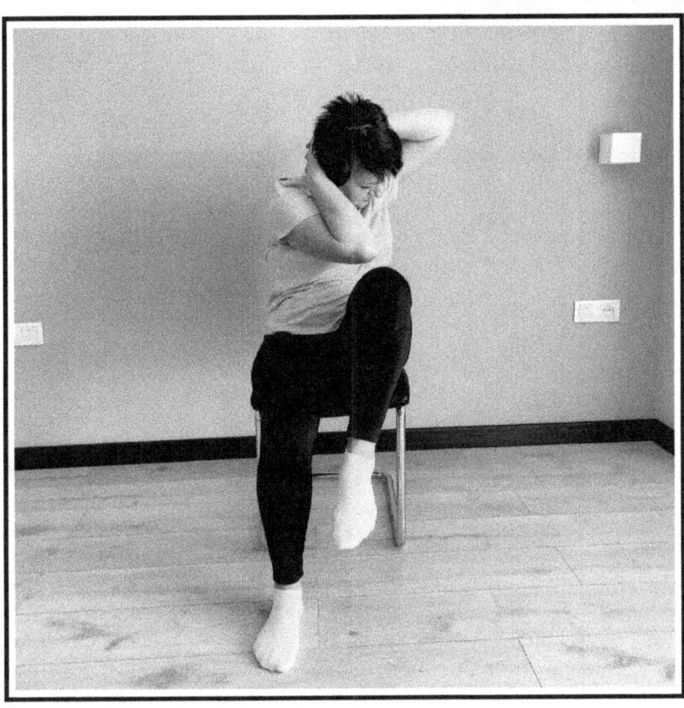

PROCEDURE:

1. Sit tall on the chair
2. Keep your knees bent
3. Put your hands behind your head
4. Inhale; engage your stomach
5. Exhale, lift your left knee and touch it with your right elbow while gently twisting your body
6. Return to the initial position
7. Alternate between sides

SUGGESTED TIPS:

- Don't hold the breath
- Don't go too fast
- Think how your abdominal muscles are getting squeezed as you do the movement slowly and with full control

Marching Arm Extensions

This is a good exercise to warm up and activate the muscles in your whole body.
It's a great fit for a warm-up exercise.

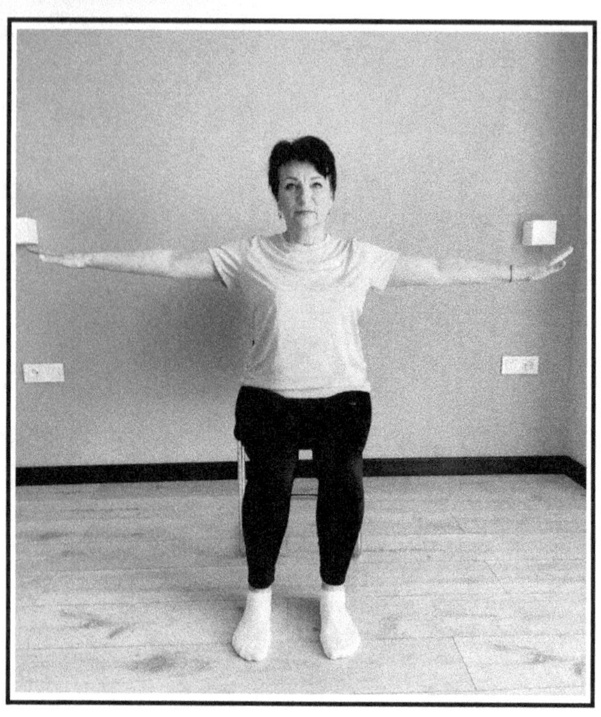 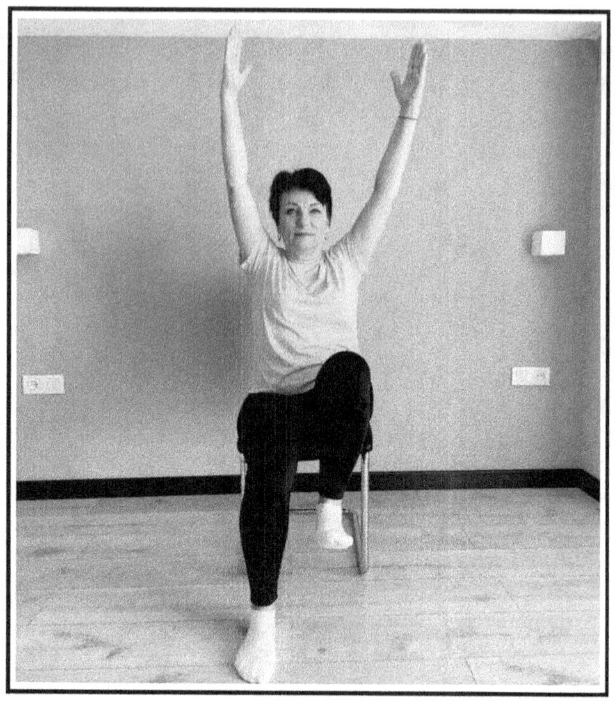

PROCEDURE:

1. Sit tall on the chair
2. Keep your knees bent
3. Put your arms out to your sides and even with your shoulders
4. Your wrists, elbows, and shoulders should be in line
5. Bring your hands up above your head; lift one of your knees up
6. Bring the knee down, and bring your arms up to your sides
7. Alternate between legs

SUGGESTED TIPS:

- Don't rush the movement
- Don't hold the breath
- Maintain regular breathing while doing this exercise

Knee Lifts

Knee Lifts are perfect for activating your hip flexor and abdominal muscles.

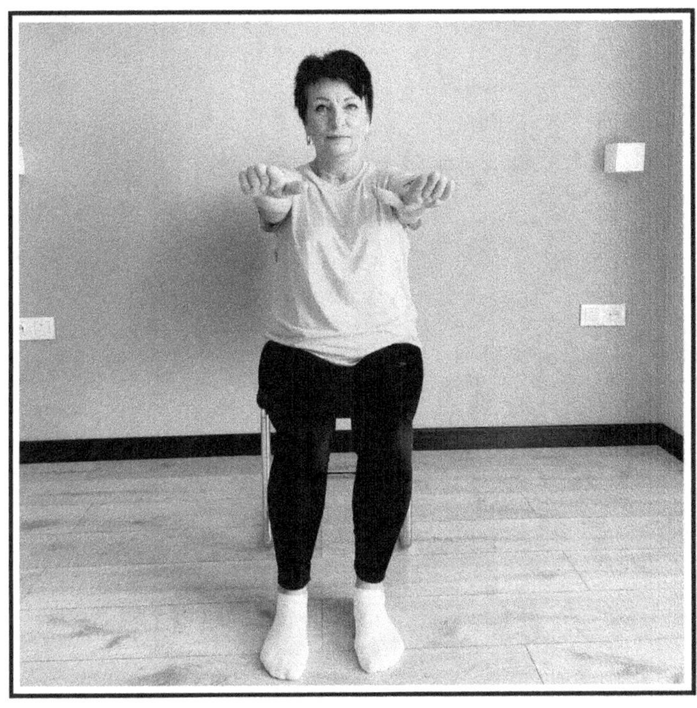 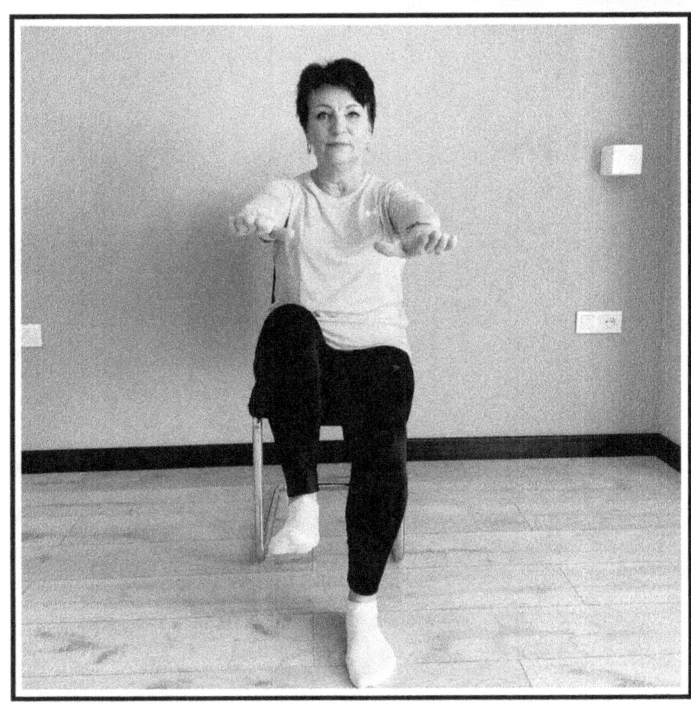

PROCEDURE:

1. Sit tall on the chair
2. Keep your knees bent
3. Extend your arms out forward
4. Inhale; squeeze your stomach muscles
5. Lift one of your knees and exhale
6. Go back to the starting position
7. Alternate between legs

SUGGESTED TIPS:

- Engage the core
- Don't hold the breath
- Think about how your abdominal muscles are getting squeezed as you do the movement slowly and with full control

47 Dynamic Cactus

Dynamic cactus is a great warm-up exercise. It moves around your lower and upper body.

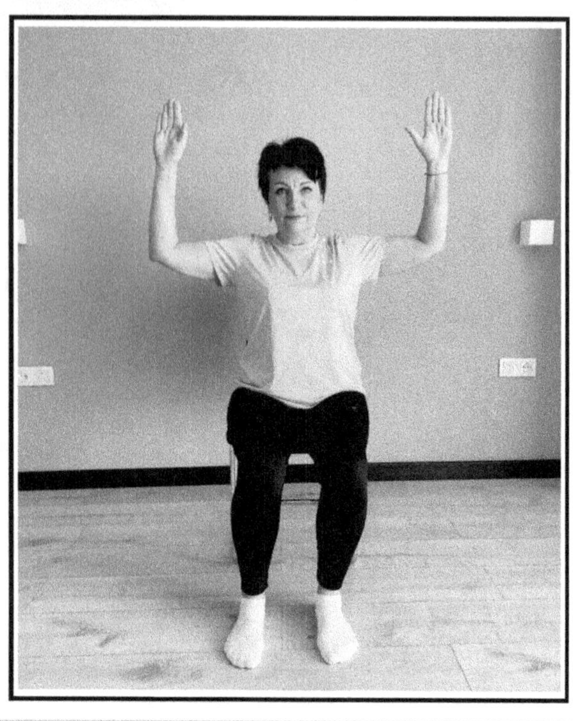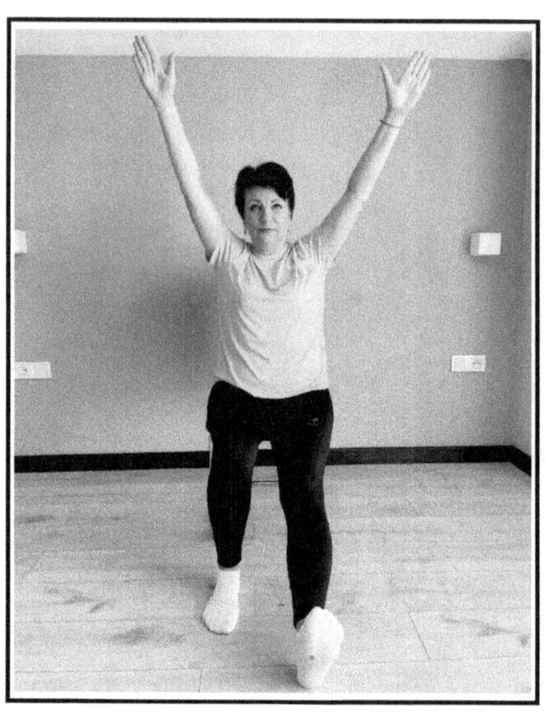

1. Sit tall on the chair
2. Keep your knees bent
3. Bring your hands next to your body at a 45-degree angle
4. Extend your arms up; take a step forward with one foot
5. Go back to the previous position
6. Extend your arms again; bring the other foot forward
7. Alternate between legs

- Don't arch the lower back
- Don't hold the breath
- Don't rush the movement
- While doing this exercise, maintain regular breathing

Seated Rope Jumps

This exercise is a fun way to warm up your shoulders.

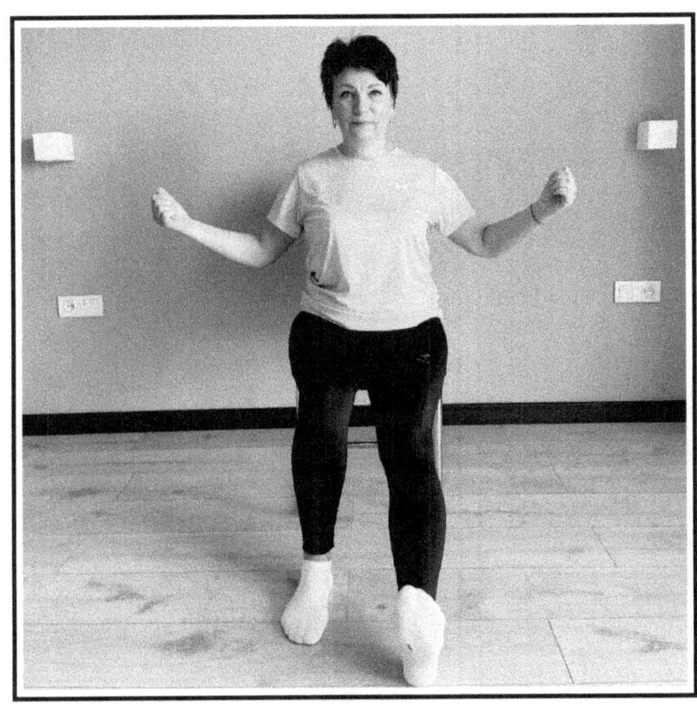
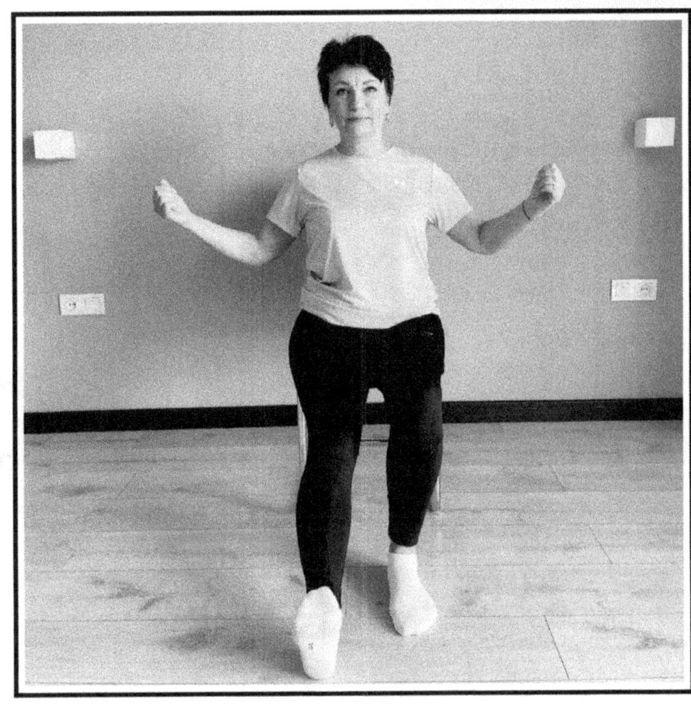

PROCEDURE:

1. Sit tall on the chair; keep your knees bent
2. Keep your arms slightly bent next to your sides
3. Start making small circles with your arms (pretend you are jumping rope)
4. While making the circles, extend one leg forward and tap the floor with your heel
5. Keep changing the legs while continuing to make the arm circles

SUGGESTED TIPS:

- Don't rush the movement
- Don't hold the breath
- While doing this exercise, maintain regular breathing

Dynamic Side Bends

Dynamic side bends stretch your big back muscles and side abdominal muscles.

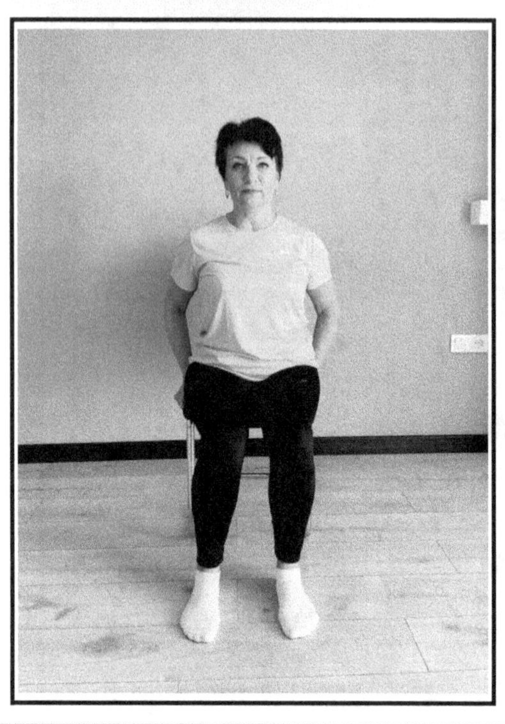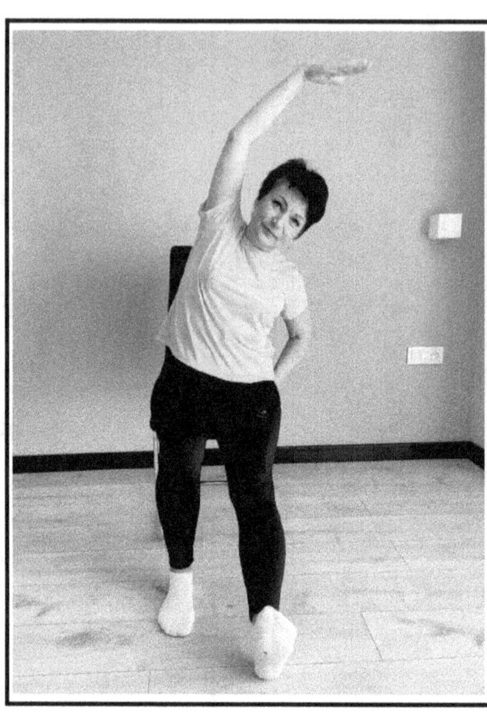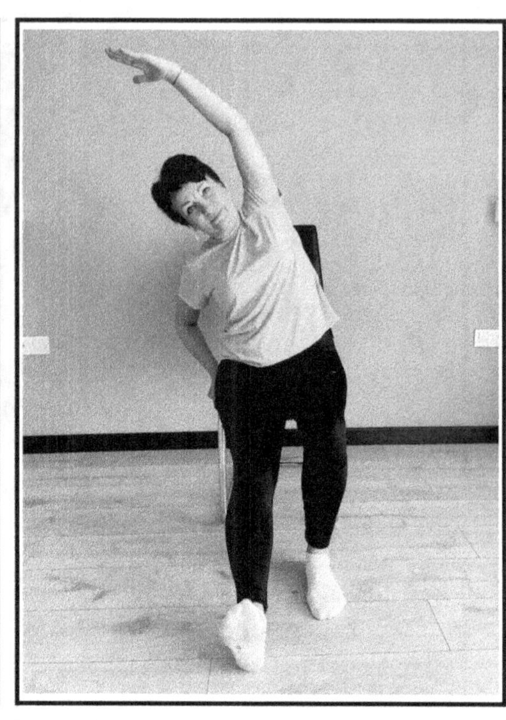

PROCEDURE:

1. Sit tall on the chair
2. Keep your knees bent
3. Keep your arms next to your body
4. Bend your body to the left side, bring your right arm up and across your head, and step forward with one foot
5. Alternate between legs

SUGGESTED TIPS:

- Don't hold the breath
- Inhale at the beginning of the movement
- Slowly exhale as you start bending your body to the side

Disco Dance (Right, Left)

Disco Dance is a great seated cardio exercise that increases the heart rate.

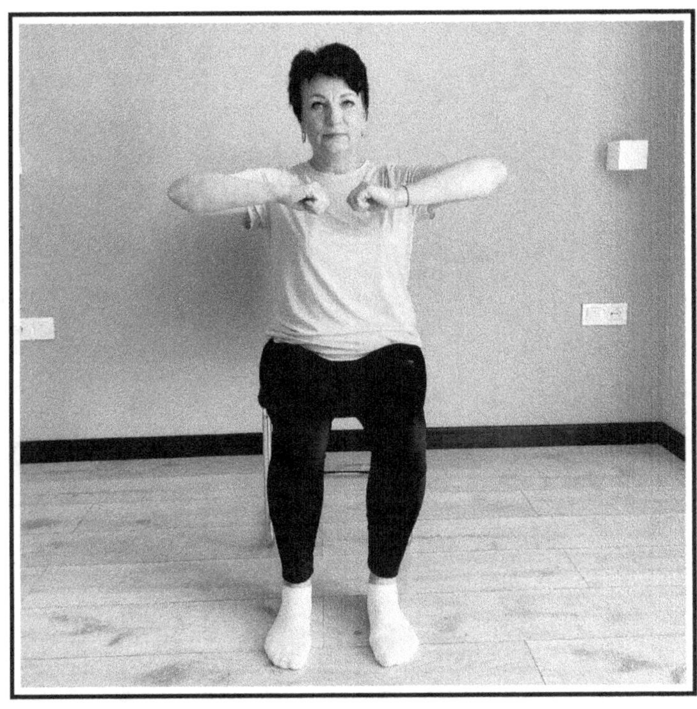 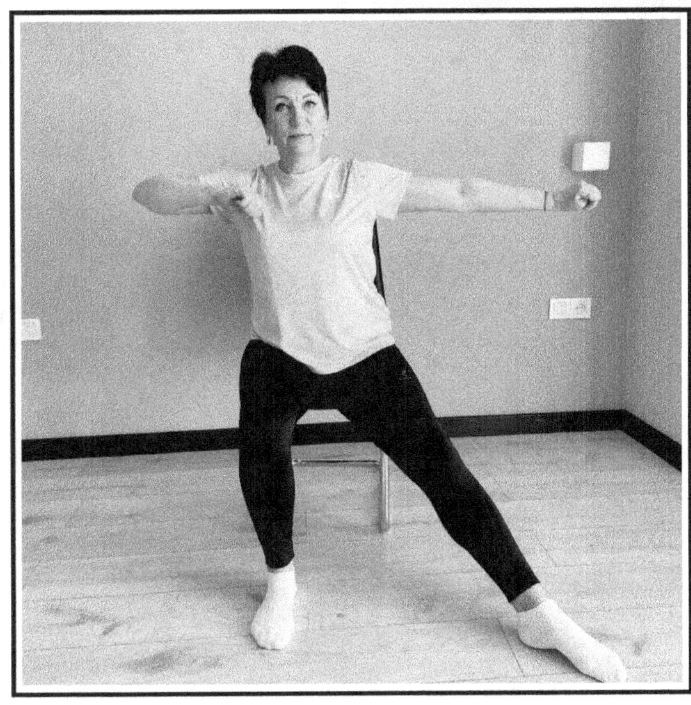

PROCEDURE:

1. Sit tall on the chair
2. Keep your knees bent
3. Bring your fists together at your chest level
4. Open your left arm and left leg to the left side
5. Bring them back; repeat the movement
6. Perform the same exercise on the left side
7. Alternate between sides

SUGGESTED TIPS:

- Don't hold the breath
- Don't do the movement slowly unless you are experiencing pain
- Maintain regular breathing while doing this exercise

51 Elbow Pull Backs

This exercise works your back muscles. It also stretches your hip flexor muscles.

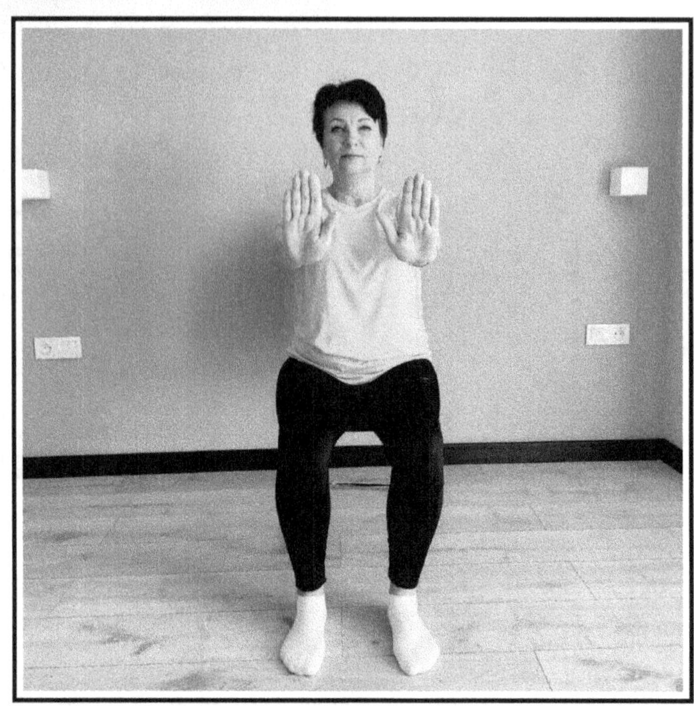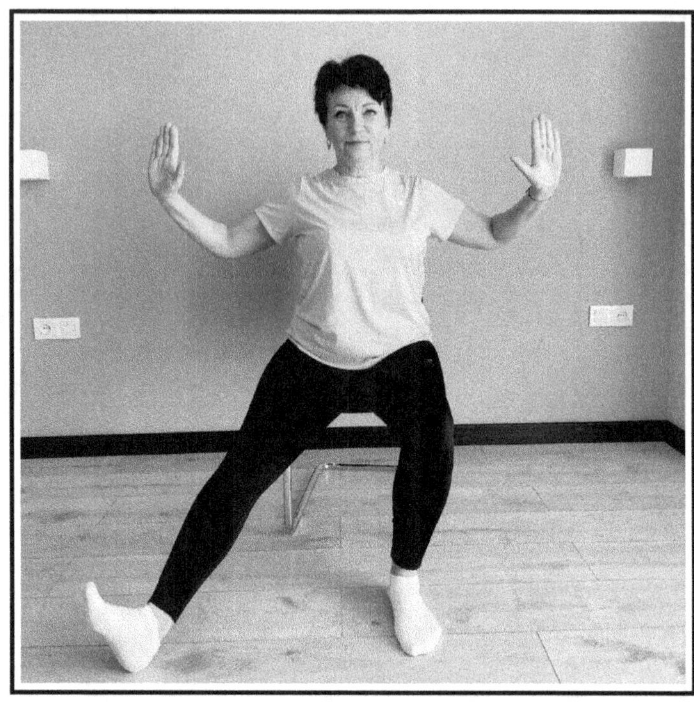

PROCEDURE:

1. Sit tall on the chair
2. Keep your knees bent
3. Extend your arms in front of you, with your palms facing forward
4. Pull your elbows backward while stretching one of your legs behind you
5. Go back to the starting position and move the other leg backward
6. Alternate between legs

SUGGESTED TIPS:

- Don't hold the breath
- Don't rush the movement
- Maintain regular breathing while doing this exercise

Hugging Leg Extension

This is a good exercise that works your quadricep muscles. It also improves your scapular (shoulder blade) health.

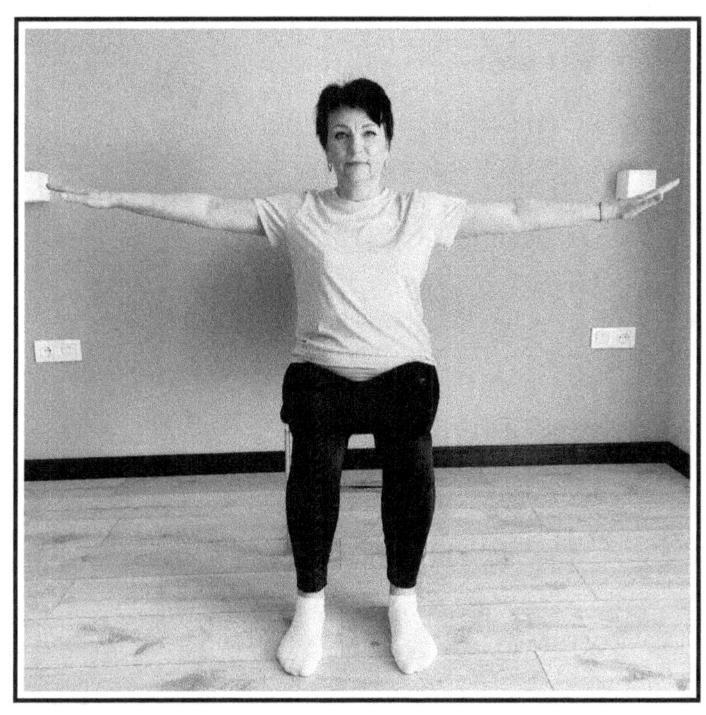 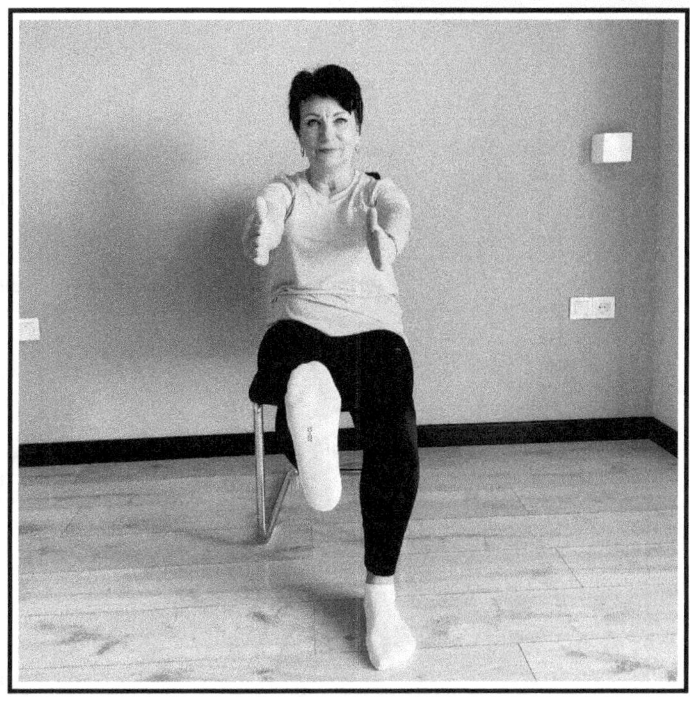

PROCEDURE:

1. Sit tall on the chair
2. Keep your knees bent
3. Keep your arms next to your sides
4. Lift your arms forward like you are about to hug a big ball
5. While you are making the movement with your hands, lift and extend your left leg
6. Go back and repeat the movement for the right leg
7. Alternate between legs

SUGGESTED TIPS:

- Don't rush the movement
- Don't hold the breath
- Inhale at the beginning of the movement
- Slowly exhale as you pretend to hug a big ball

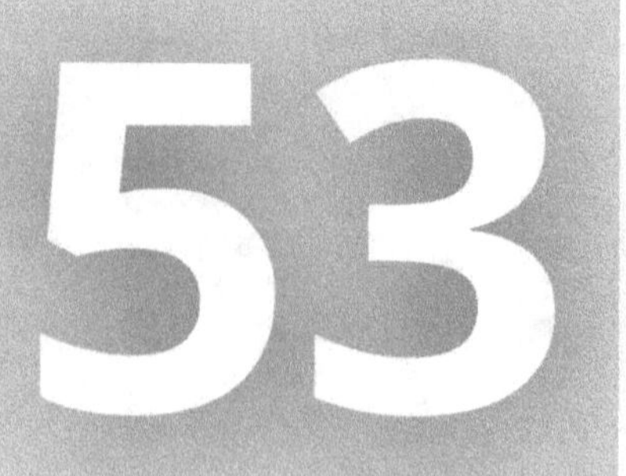

53

Dynamic Chest Fly

This exercise dynamically warms up your chest muscles and moves your body.

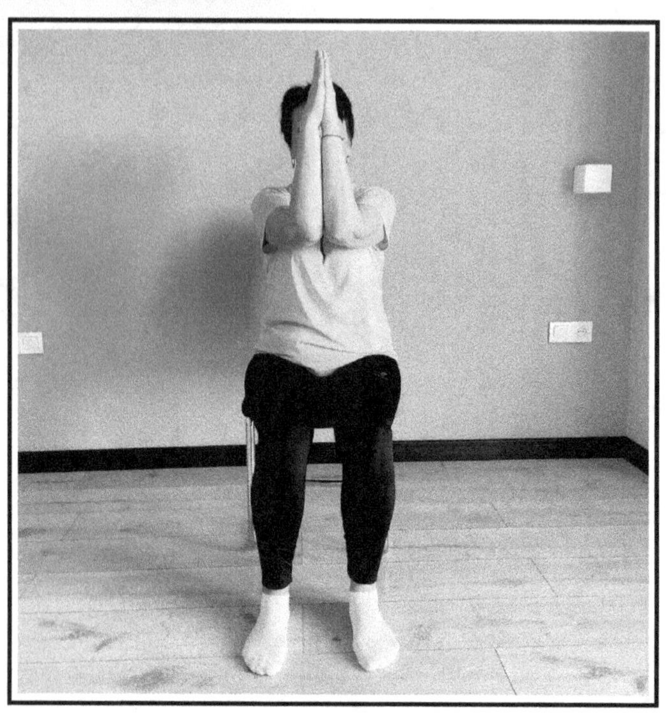 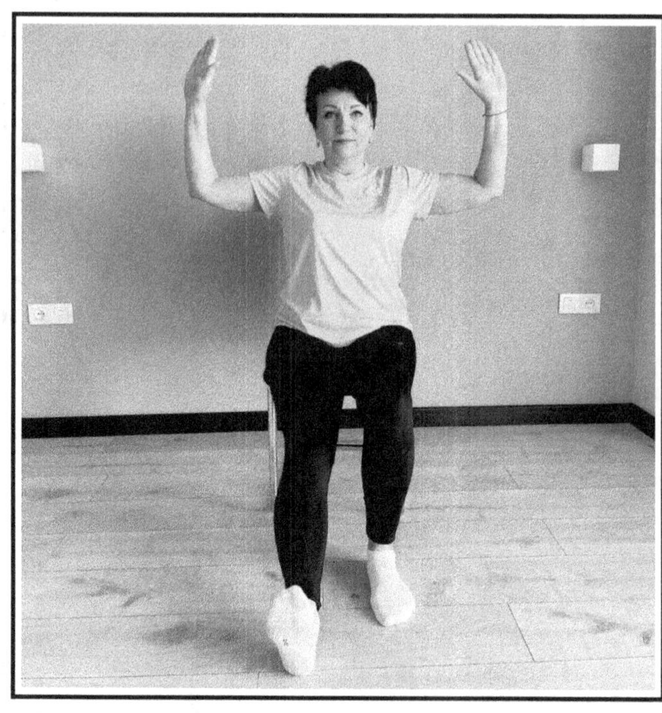

PROCEDURE:

1. Sit tall on the chair; keep your knees bent
2. Bend your arms at the elbow and elevate them at a 90-degree angle
3. Bring your elbows and forearms together
4. While doing that, step with one foot forward
5. Bring your hands and leg to the initial position
6. Repeat the exercise alternating between legs

SUGGESTED TIPS:

- Don't arch the lower back
- Don't hold the breath
- Don't rush the movement
- Maintain regular breathing while doing this exercise

Exercises with Extra Weight

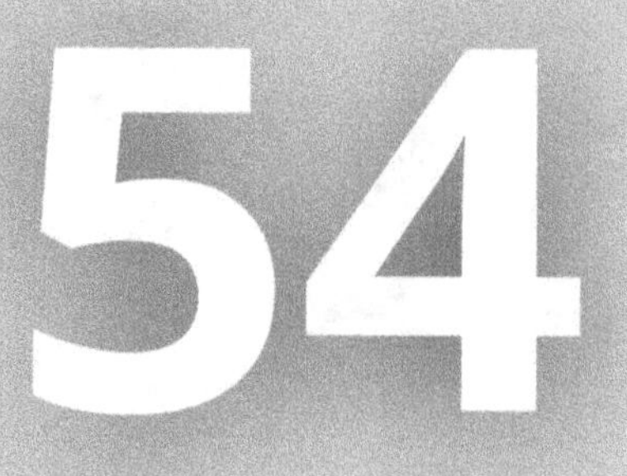

54 Front Raises

Front Raises isolate your shoulder muscles.

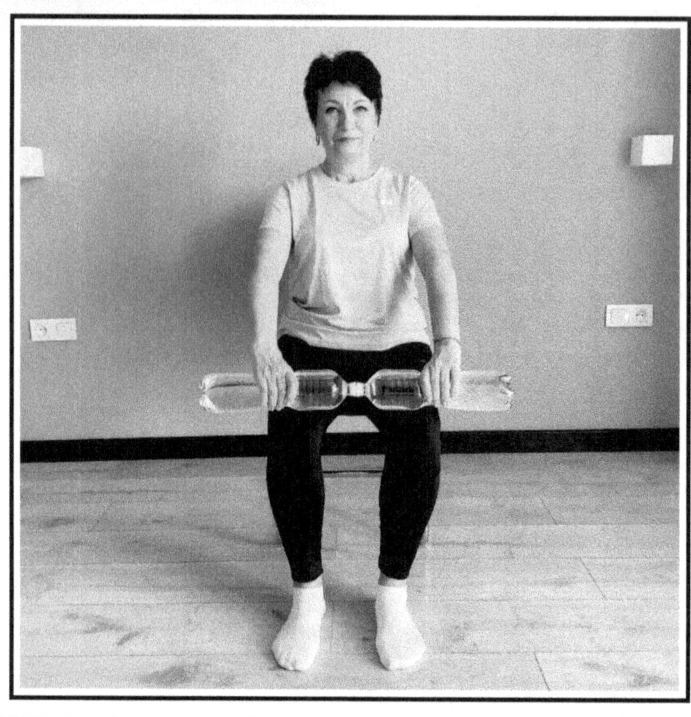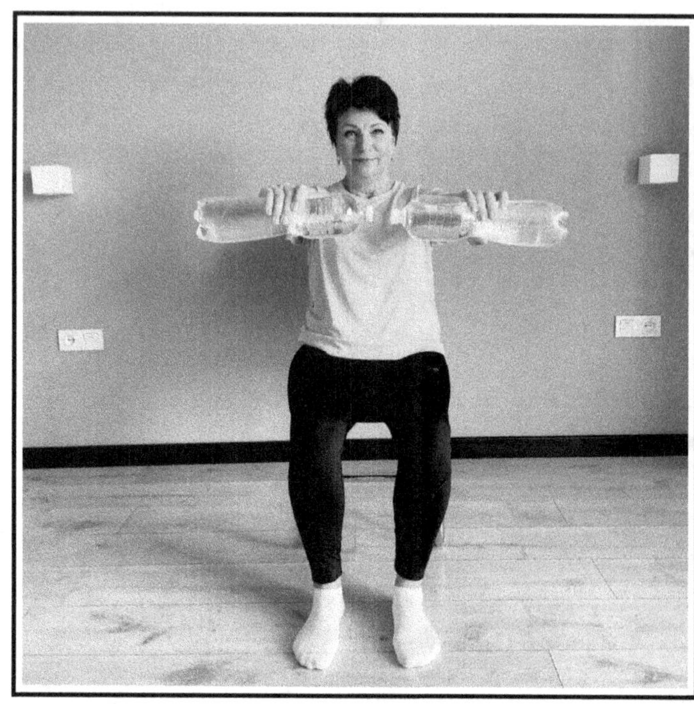

1. Sit tall on the chair; keep your knees bent
2. Hold the bottles in your hands; inhale
3. Exhale and lift your arms forward
4. The bottles should be at eye level
5. Slowly lower the bottles to the starting position
6. Repeat the movement

SUGGESTED TIPS:

- Keep your elbows fully extended
- Don't rush the movement
- Don't go too high up
- Don't hold the breath
- Follow the tempo of this exercise (i.e., medium – not too fast or too slow)

PAGE 76

Biceps Curls

Biceps Curls are a phenomenal exercise that activates your bicep muscles. It's a good exercise to strengthen and develop your arm muscles.

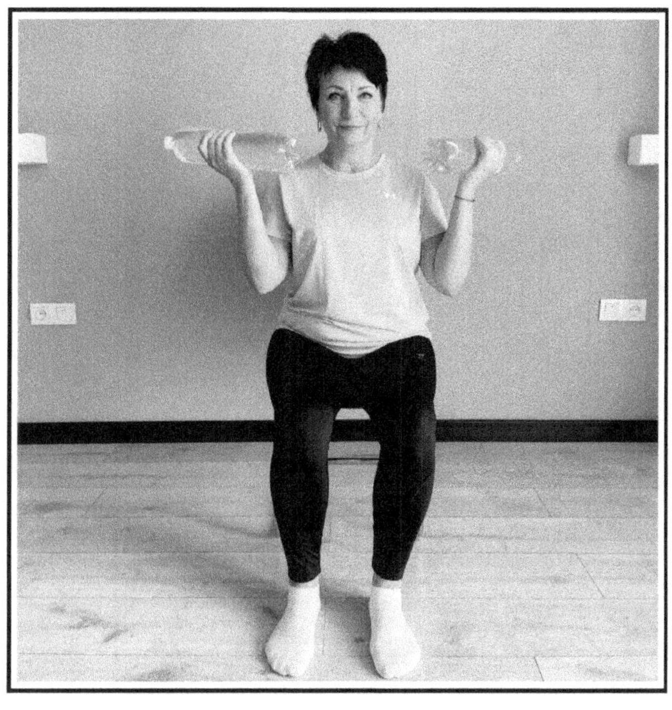
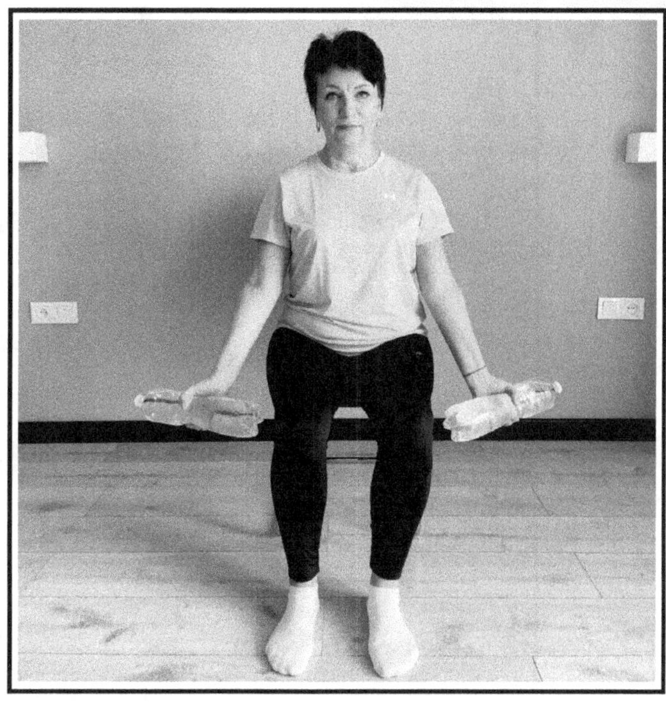

PROCEDURE:

1. Sit tall on the chair; keep your knees bent
2. Hold the bottles in your hands with the elbows closely to your sides; inhale
3. Exhale and bend your elbows
4. Slowly lower the bottles until your elbows are almost fully extended
5. Repeat the movement

SUGGESTED TIPS:

- Don't rush the movement
- Properly extend the elbows
- Don't hold the breath
- Do this exercise with full control
- Feel your biceps getting contracted

56 Shoulder Presses

Shoulder Presses are one of the best exercises to strengthen your shoulder muscles. This exercise also works your triceps, back, and core muscles.

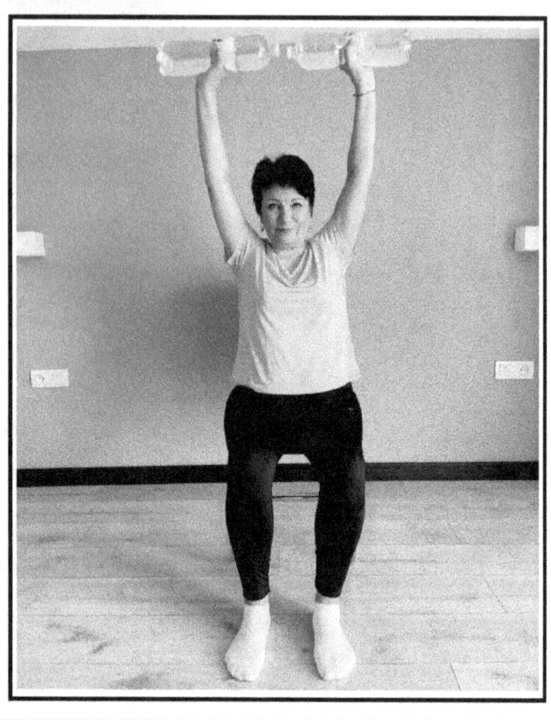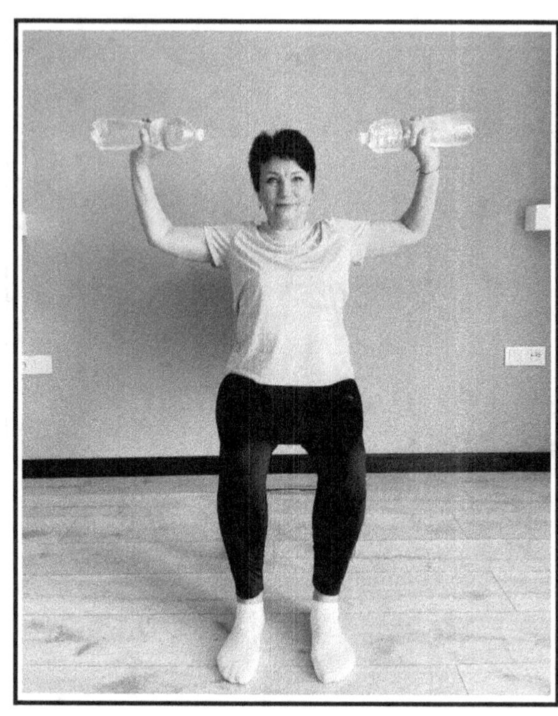

PROCEDURE:

1. Sit tall on the chair; keep your knees bent
2. Hold the bottles in your hands
3. Bend your elbows and place them at your sides (the bottles should be at ear level); inhale
4. Then exhale and press the bottles up, making sure your arms are fully extended
5. Slowly lower the bottles to your ear level; repeat the movement

SUGGESTED TIPS:

- Don't keep your elbows spread outward to the side
- Don't hold the breath; extend your arms fully
- Don't lower the dumbbells underneath the ear level
- Keep your elbows a little bit tucked in this exercise (spreading them outward to the side can damage the shoulder capsule, the membrane around your shoulder)

Back Rows

This exercise works your back muscles. It also targets your quadricep muscles.

57

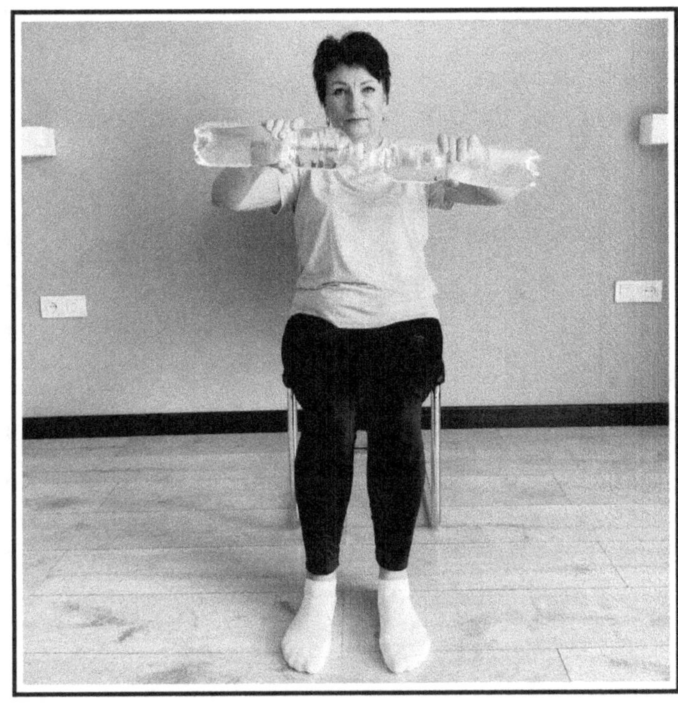 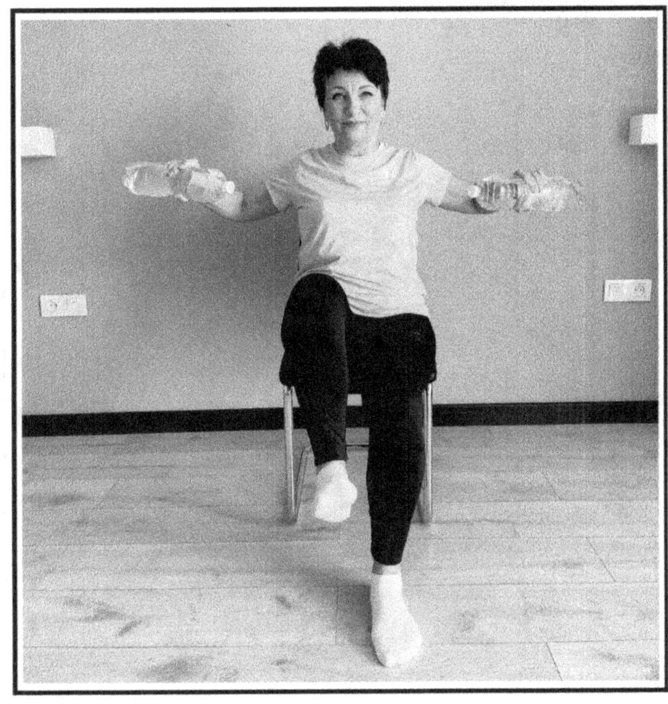

PROCEDURE:

1. Sit tall on the chair; keep your knees bent
2. Hold the bottles in your hands at chest level; inhale
3. Exhale, and row the bottles backward, while lifting your left knee up
4. Go to the initial position
5. Repeat the movement alternating between legs

SUGGESTED TIPS:

- Don't hold the breath
- Don't row too fast
- Follow the tempo of this exercise (i.e., medium – not too fast or too slow)

58 Chest Presses

Chest Presses are great for developing your triceps, shoulders, and chest. They also activate your quadricep muscles.

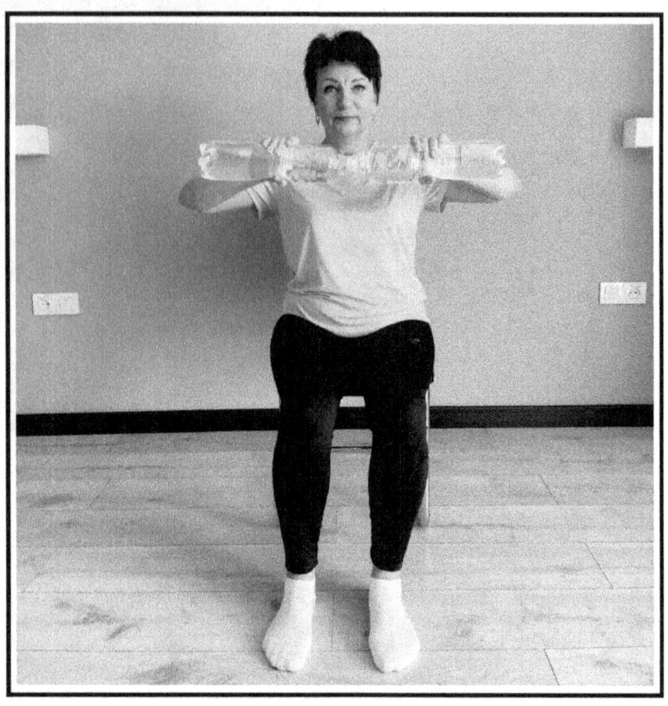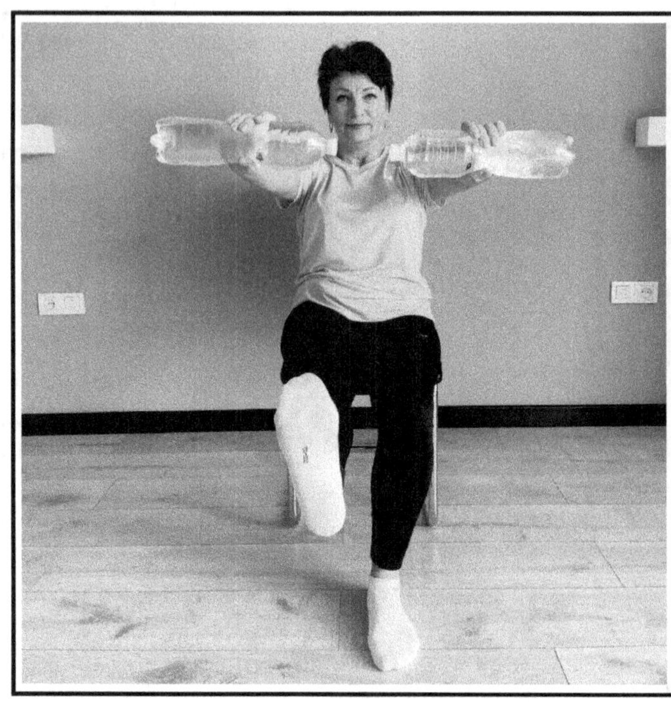

1. Sit tall on the chair
2. Keep your knees bent
3. Hold the bottles in your hands at chest level; inhale
4. Exhale, and press the bottles forward, while extending your left leg forward
5. Go to the initial position
6. Repeat the movement alternating between legs

- Don't hold the breath
- Don't press too fast
- Don't rush while doing the exercise
- Follow the tempo of this exercise (i.e., medium – not too fast or too slow)

PAGE 80

Triceps Extension

Triceps Extensions are one of the best exercises for strengthening all three heads of the triceps muscle. It also strengthens your elbows.

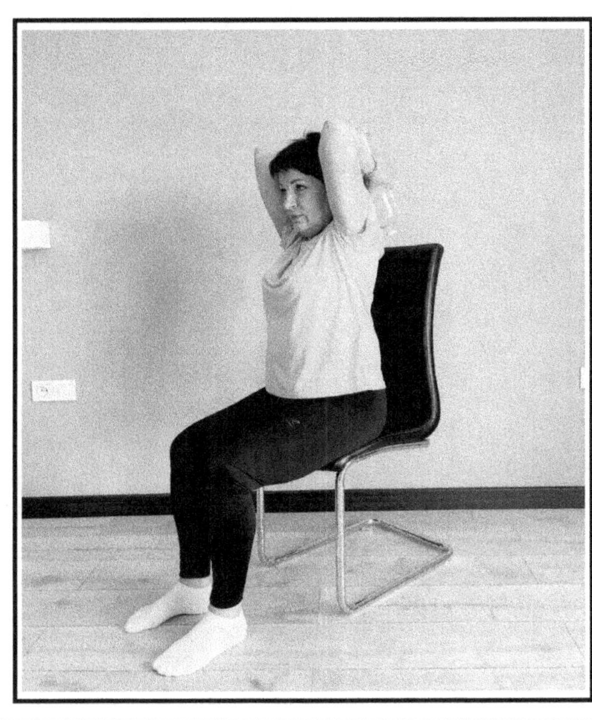

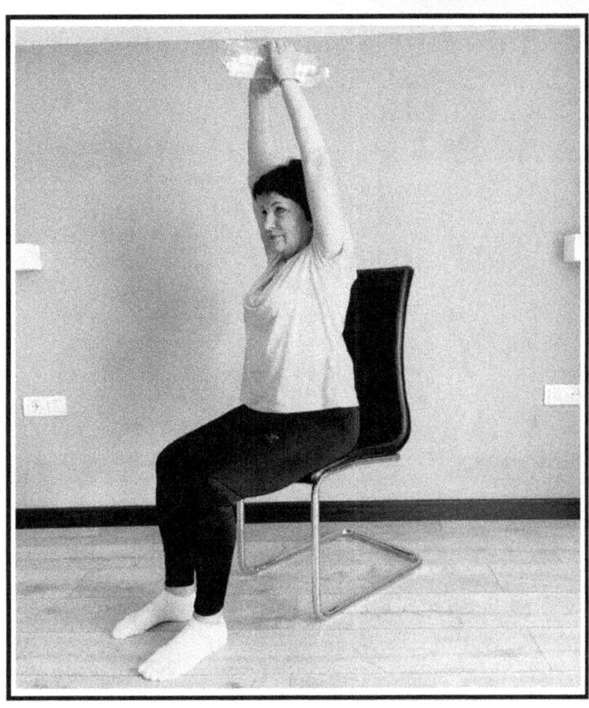

PROCEDURE:

1. Sit a bit forward on the chair; keep your knees bent
2. Hold the bottle in your hands
3. With your elbows bent, bring the bottle behind your head
4. Keep your elbows close to your head; inhale
5. Exhale and extend your arms up as much as you can
6. Slowly lower the bottle while bending your elbows
7. Repeat the movement

SUGGESTED TIPS:

- Extend your elbows
- Don't rush the movement
- Don't hold the breath
- Do this exercise with full control
- Feel your triceps getting stretched

60 Seated Bent Over Row

This is a popular exercise for building the latissimus dorsi (lat muscles)of the back.

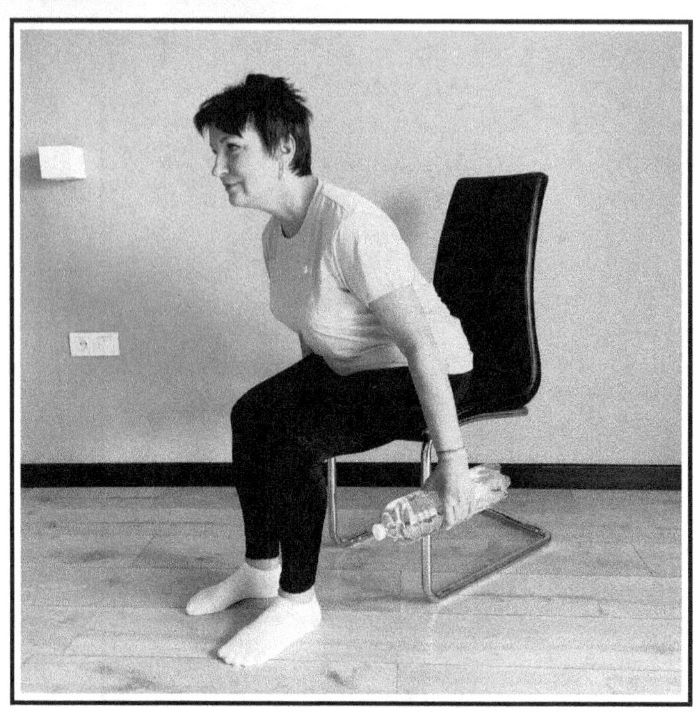

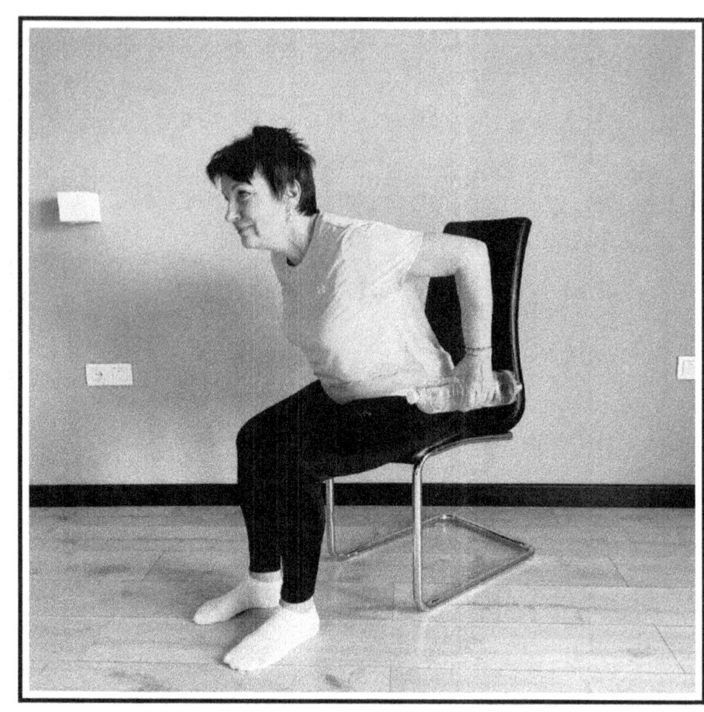

PROCEDURE:

1. Sit a bit forward on the chair; keep your knees bent
2. Hold the bottles in your hands next to your thighs
3. Bend your body forward; inhale
4. Start the movement with your shoulder blades and pull the bottles up to waist level
5. Exhale, slowly return to the starting position
6. Repeat the movement

SUGGESTED TIPS:

- Don't rush the movement
- Don't hold the breath
- Be in full control
- Feel your lat muscles getting contracted

PAGE 82

Shoulder Raises (Right, Left)

Shoulder Raises are a perfect exercise that improves your shoulder strength. They also work your back muscles.

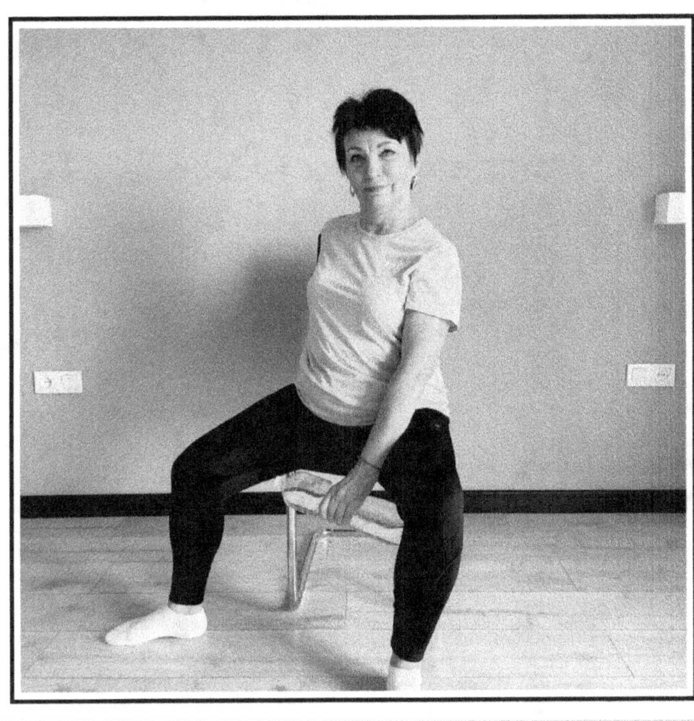

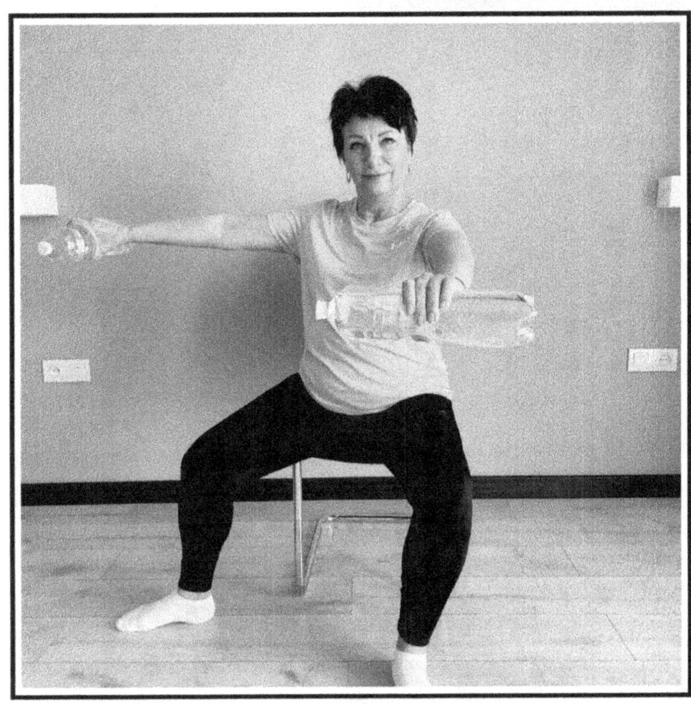

PROCEDURE:

1. Sit tall on the chair
2. Keep your knees bent and open to the side
3. Hold the bottles in your hands
4. Put your left hand in front of you on the chair, and put your right hand to your side; inhale
5. Exhale, and lift your left arm forward and your right arm sideways
6. Slowly control the weight on the way down
7. Alternate between sides

SUGGESTED TIPS:

- Don't hold the breath; don't use momentum
- Don't bend your elbows
- Don't rush while doing this exercise
- Follow the tempo of this exercise (i.e., medium – not too fast or too slow)

Stretches

Seated Neck Stretch
(Right, Left)

This is a great way to stretch and relax your neck muscles, especially after a long day at the office.

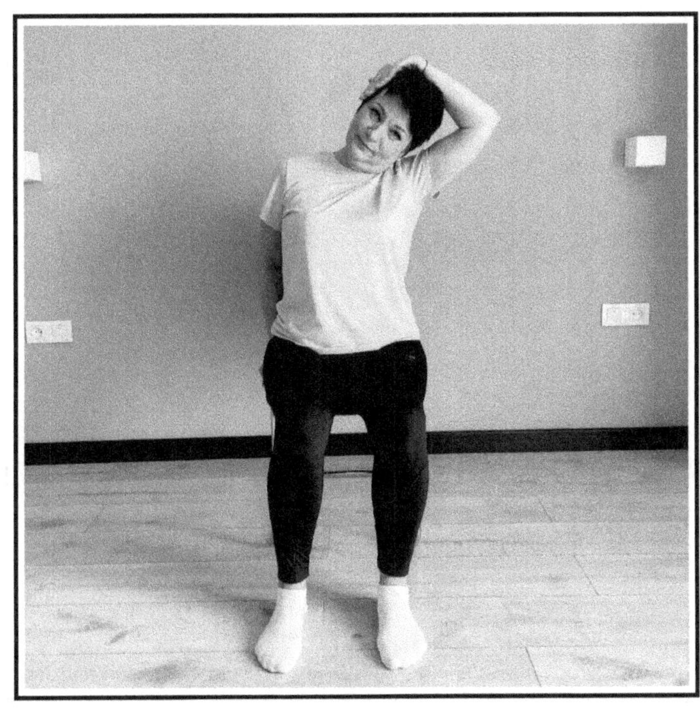

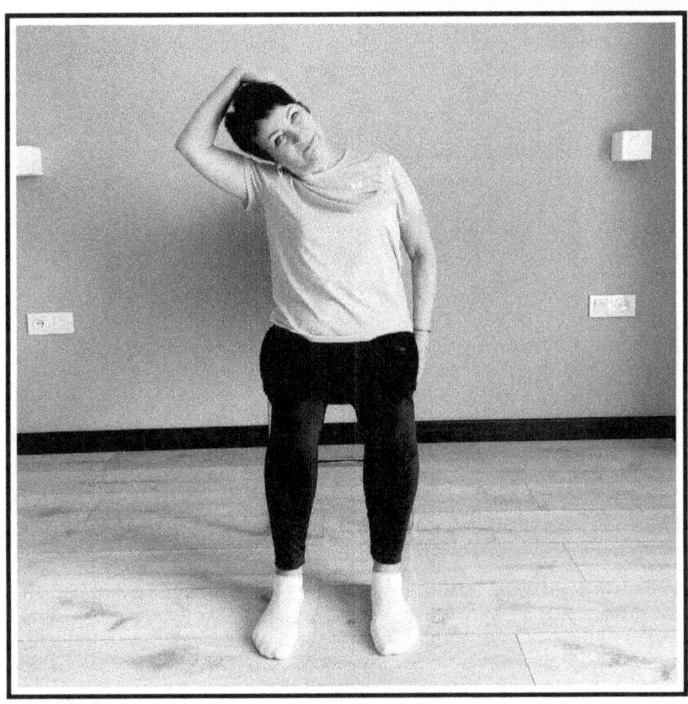

PROCEDURE:

1. Sit on the chair with your posture tall
2. Lift your arms up and put the left hand on the head
3. Grab the chair with your right hand
4. Look up and gently press your head to your left shoulder
5. Hold the stretch
6. Perform the same exercise with the other hand

SUGGESTED TIPS:

- Don't push the neck too hard
- As you stretch the neck, take a deep breath and slowly exhale

63 Cross-Body Shoulder Stretch
(Right, Left)

This exercise gives you an incredible stretch in your side shoulders. It stretches your back muscles as well.

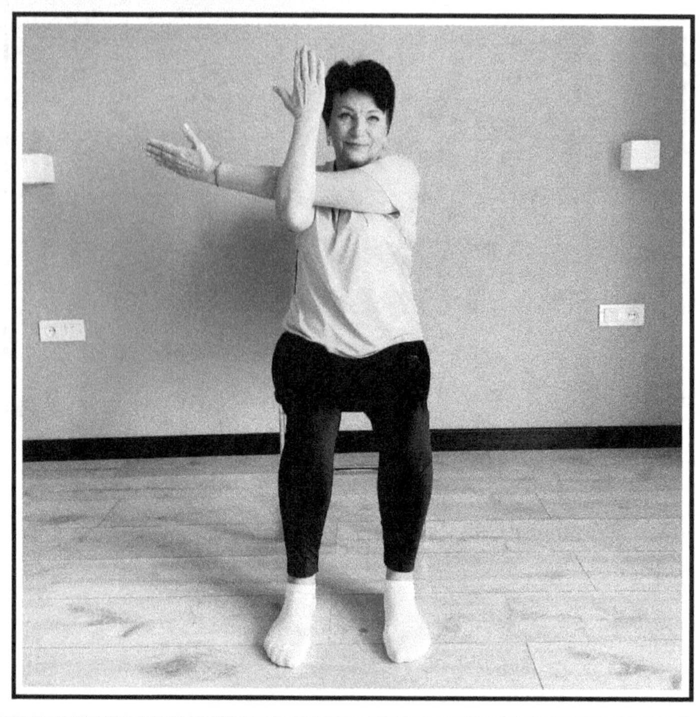 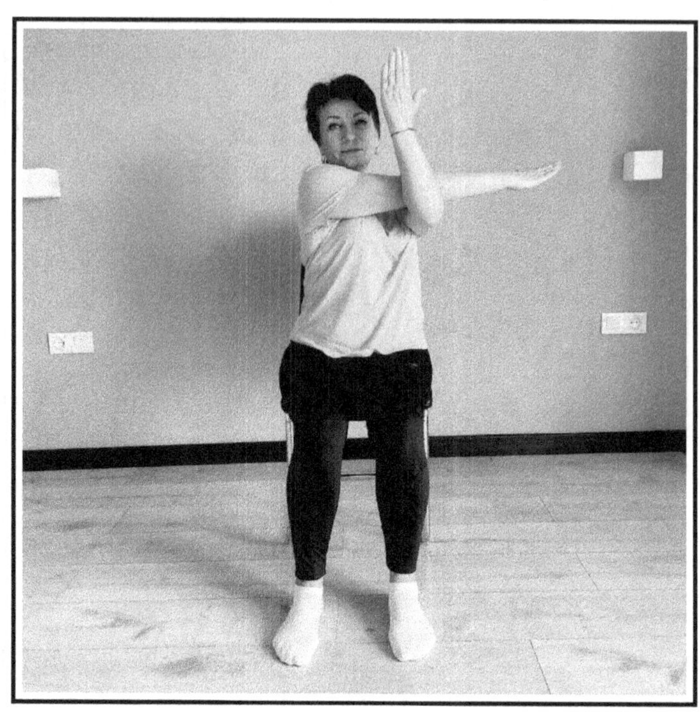

PROCEDURE:

1. Sit tall on the chair
2. Keep your knees bent
3. Lift your right arm across the body
4. With your left forearm, push your right arm even more across the body
5. Hold the stretch and maintain regular breathing
6. Perform the same exercise with the right hand

SUGGESTED TIPS:

- Don't feel the stretch
- Don't hold the breath
- Once you start feeling the stretch in your shoulders, hold that static position before moving to the other arm

Hamstring Stretch
(Right, Left)

This is a phenomenal exercise that increases your hamstring and calf flexibility.

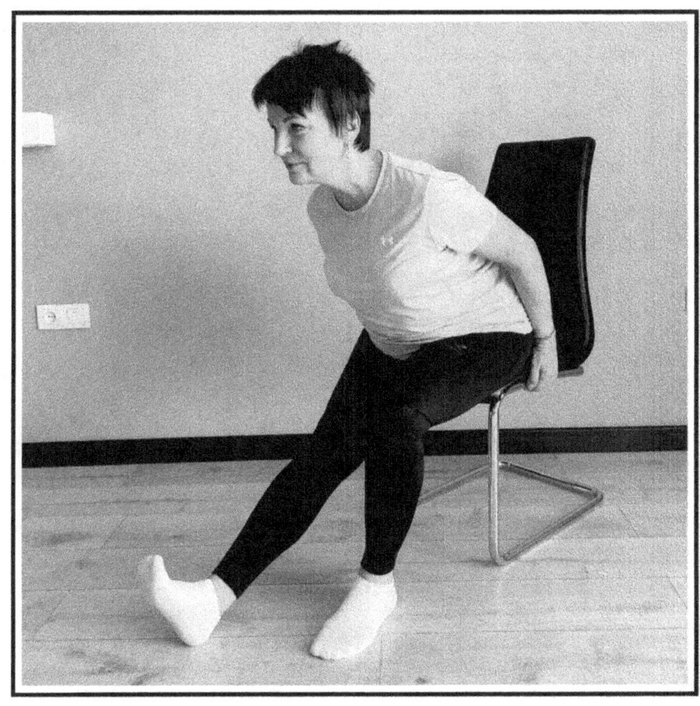

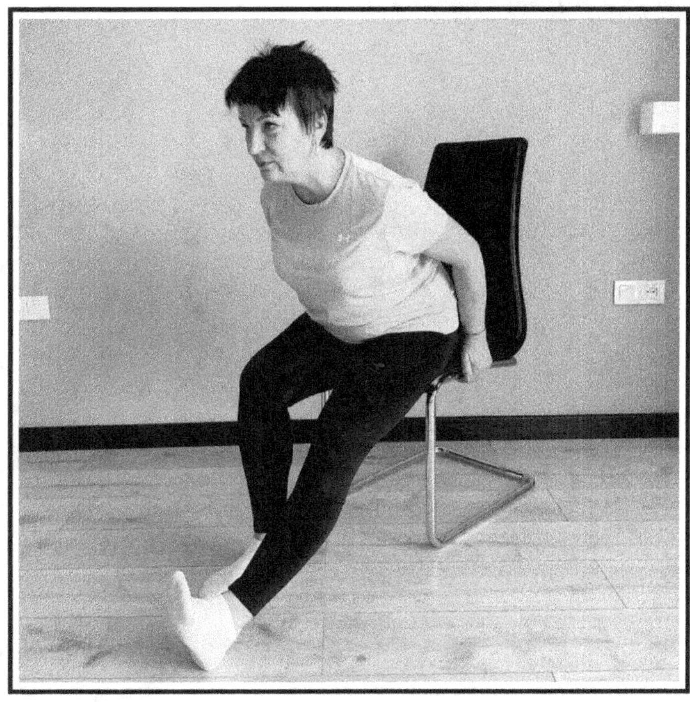

PROCEDURE:

1. Sit tall on the chair
2. Straighten your right leg, keep the left leg bent
3. Point your right toes up; inhale
4. Exhale and lean your body forward
5. Hold the stretch
6. Perform the same exercise with your right leg bent

SUGGESTED TIPS:

- Don't bend the knee
- Point the toes up
- Don't arch the lower back
- Don't hold the breath
- Don't rush when leaning your body forward
- Perform this exercise slowly with full control

Contraction and Release

This exercise stretches your mid-back muscles. It also serves as a good reminder to have good posture whenever you are in a sitting position.

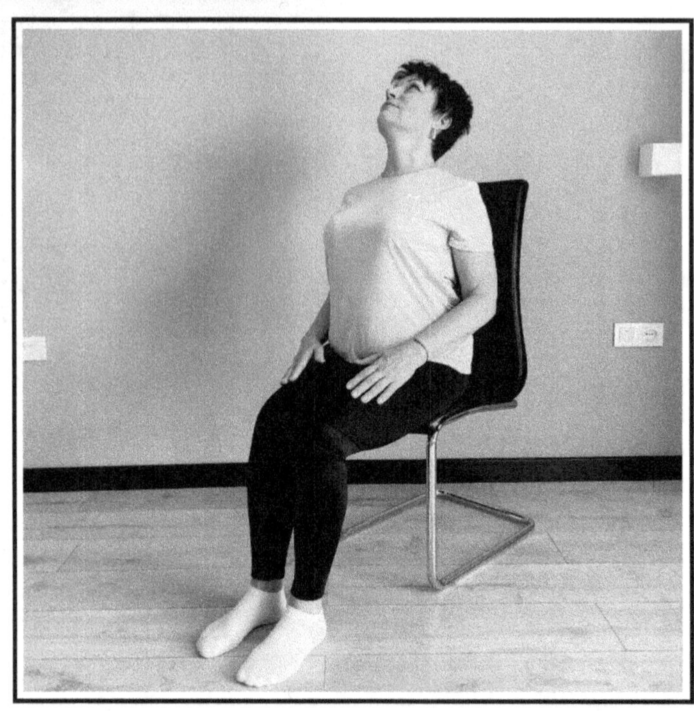 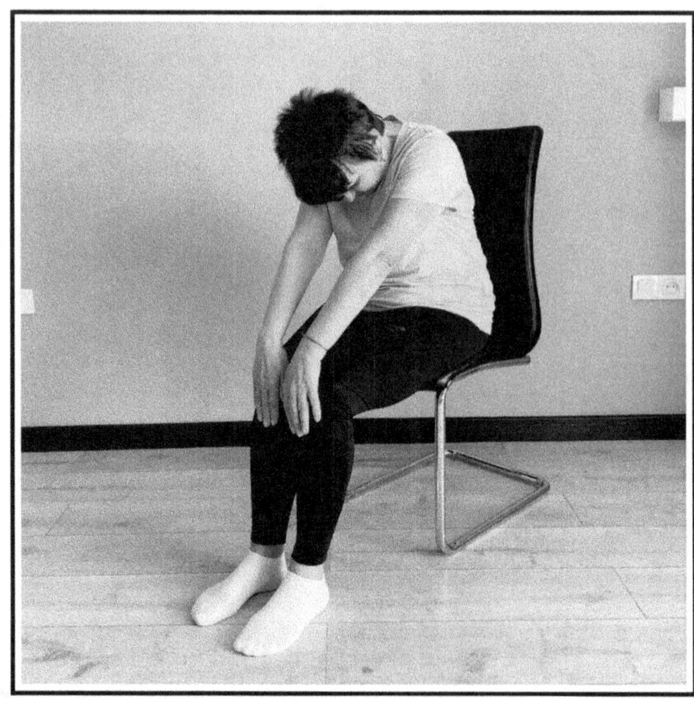

PROCEDURE:

1. Sit on the chair with your posture tall
2. Start rounding the spine
3. Let your head slightly drop forward
4. Extend your spine to the starting position
5. Repeat the movement

SUGGESTED TIPS:

- Don't rush the movement
- As you bend forward, take a deep breath and slowly exhale

Seated Upper-Body Stretch

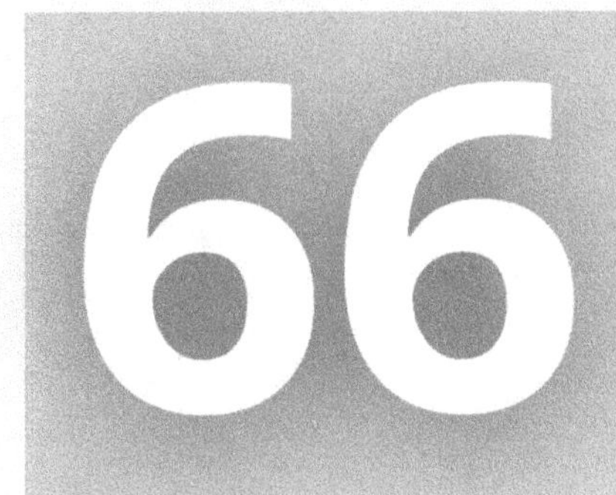

This exercise improves your thoracic mobility; it stretches your latissimus and external oblique abdominal muscles.

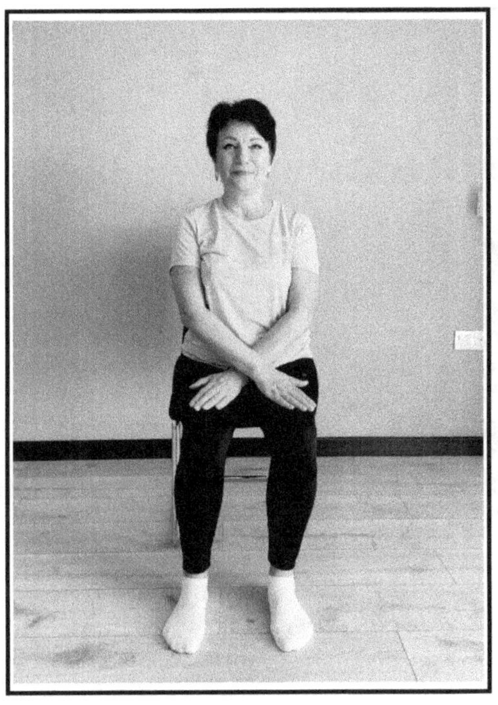
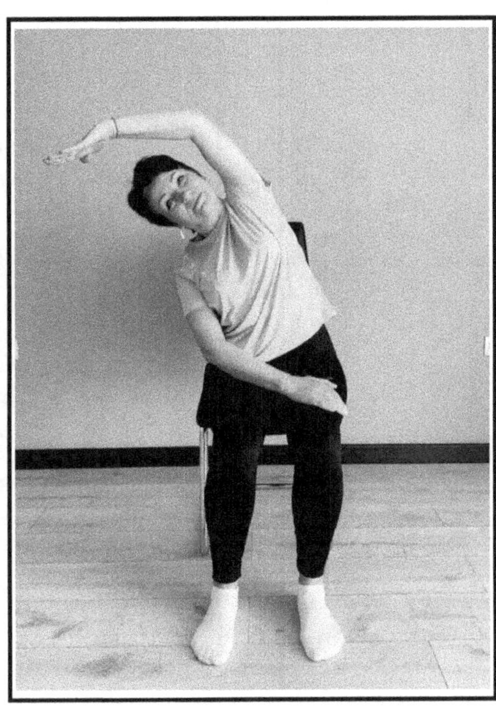
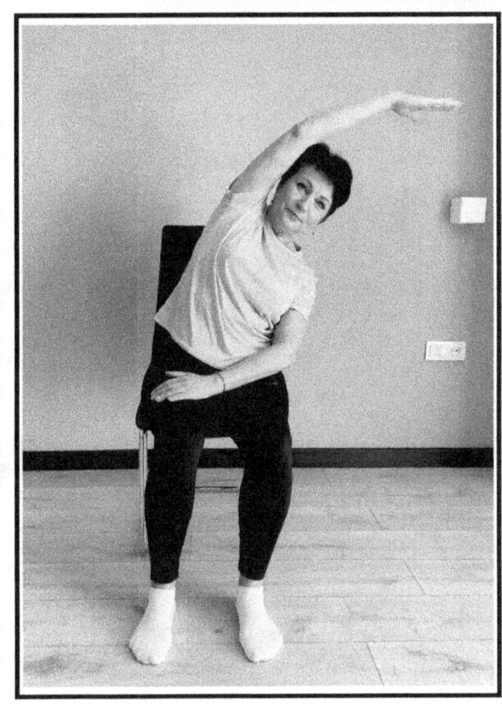

PROCEDURE:

1. Sit on the chair
2. Lift your arm up and across your head; bend your body to the side
3. Come back to the starting position and rotate to the side
4. Alternate between sides

SUGGESTED TIPS:

- Don't rush the movement
- Inhale and exhale as you are rotating to the side

67 Neck & Arm Stretch
(Right, Left)

This is an amazing exercise that stretches your neck, forearms, and hands.

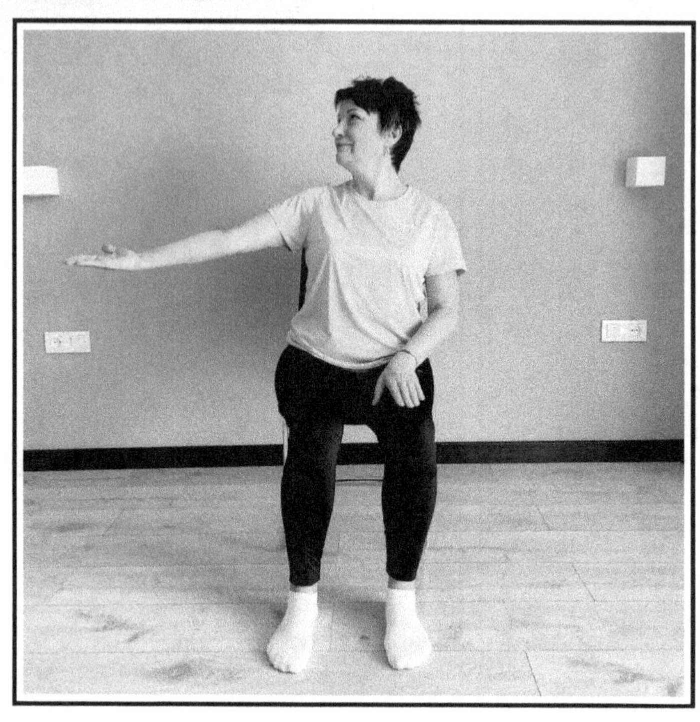 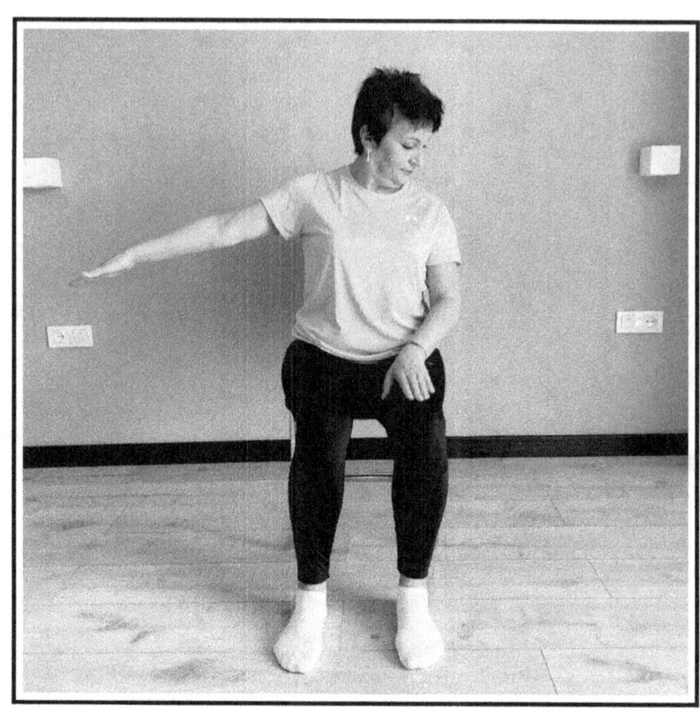

PROCEDURE:

1. Sit tall on the chair; keep your knees bent
2. Reach out with your right arm to the side and spread your fingers wide
3. Gently bend your neck to the left
4. Inhale, turn your palm up, and gently lift your chin up
5. Exhale and bring your palm and chin down
6. Repeat the exercise

SUGGESTED TIPS:

- Don't rush the movement
- Don't hold the breath
- Feel the stretch as you do the steps slowly and in control

Shoulder Twist

The shoulder twist is a fantastic exercise that stretches your mid-back muscles.

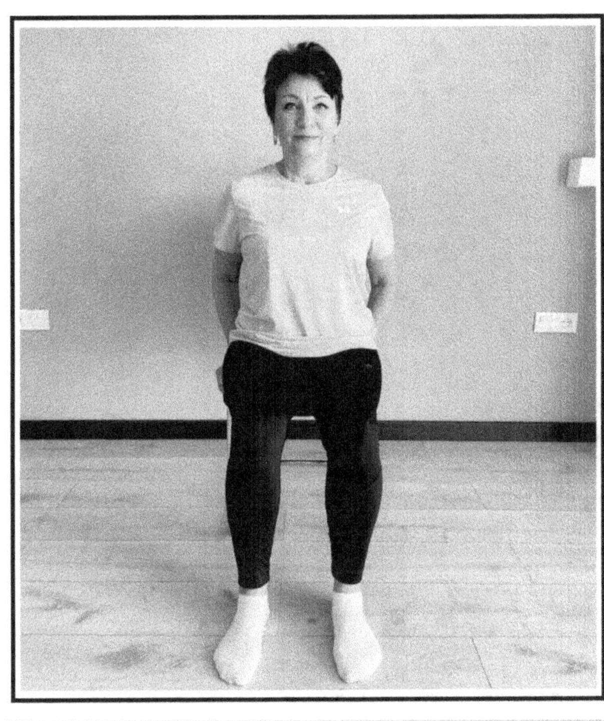 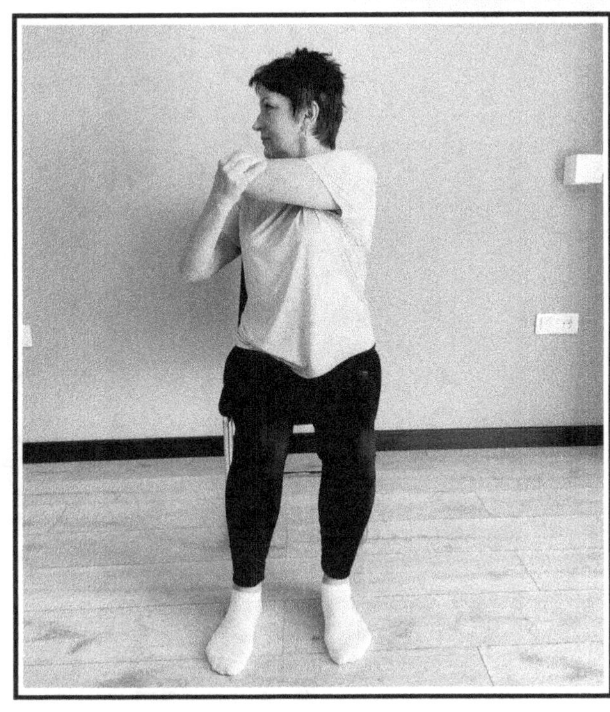

PROCEDURE:

1. Sit tall on the chair; keep your knees bent
2. Put your left hand on the right shoulder
3. Keep your elbows away from your body and inhale
4. With your right hand, grab your left elbow and pull to the right side
5. Hold the stretch and exhale
6. Do the other side as well

SUGGESTED TIPS:

- Don't do one side only
- Don't hold the breath
- Don't go too fast
- Hold the shoulder twist position for 5-8 breaths
- Then change sides, and do the same number of breaths

69 Chair Hero Pose

This exercise improves your breathing and supplies your brain and body with more oxygen.

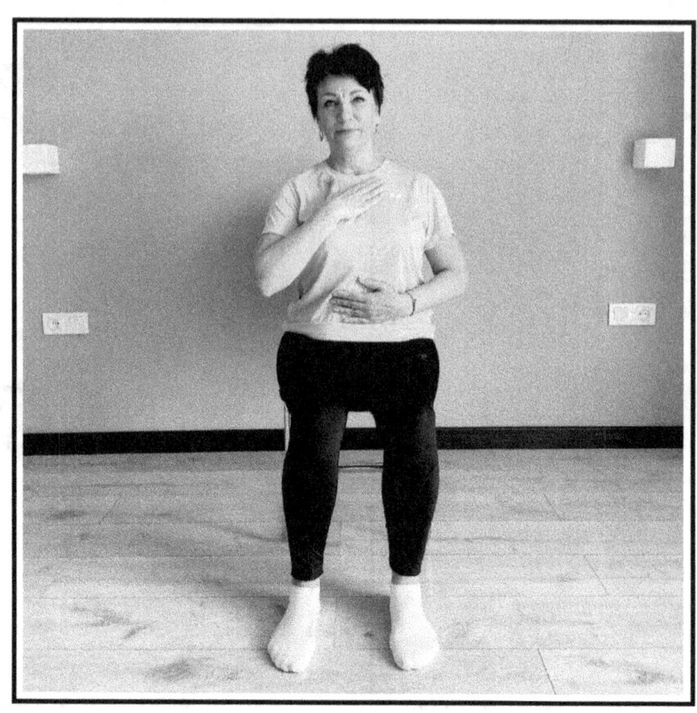

PROCEDURE:

1. Sit on the chair with your posture tall
2. Put one hand on the chest and the other hand on the stomach
3. Take a deep breath through the nose and expand your chest
4. Slowly exhale
5. Make sure you are not breathing from the stomach
6. Keep breathing

SUGGESTED TIPS:

- Don't breathe through the stomach
- Make sure to do this exercise in a quiet place (e.g., lower the music or amount of external noise)
- Focus on your breath

Exercises for Arthritis

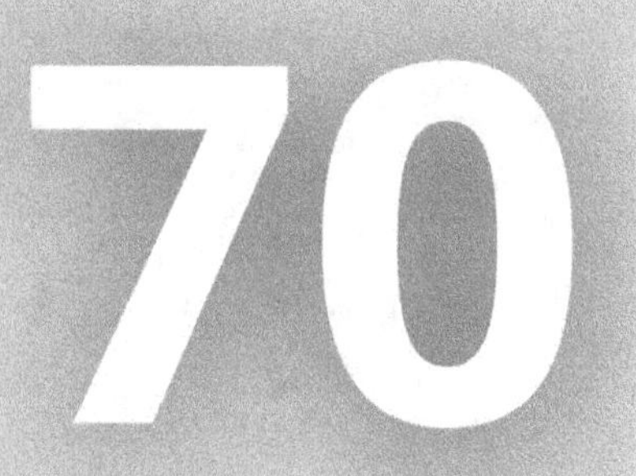

70 Wrist Flexion and Extension

This exercise helps strengthen your forearm and wrist muscles. It will also improve wrist flexibility.

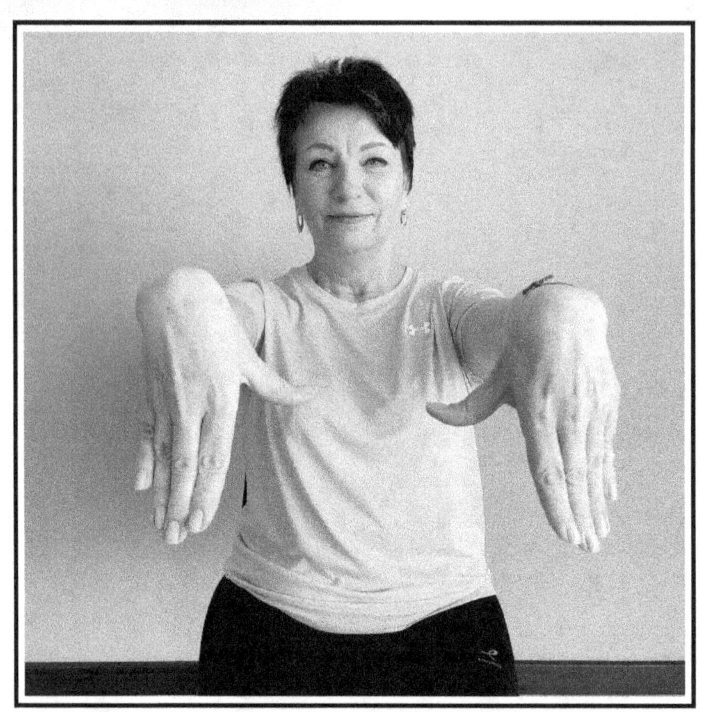

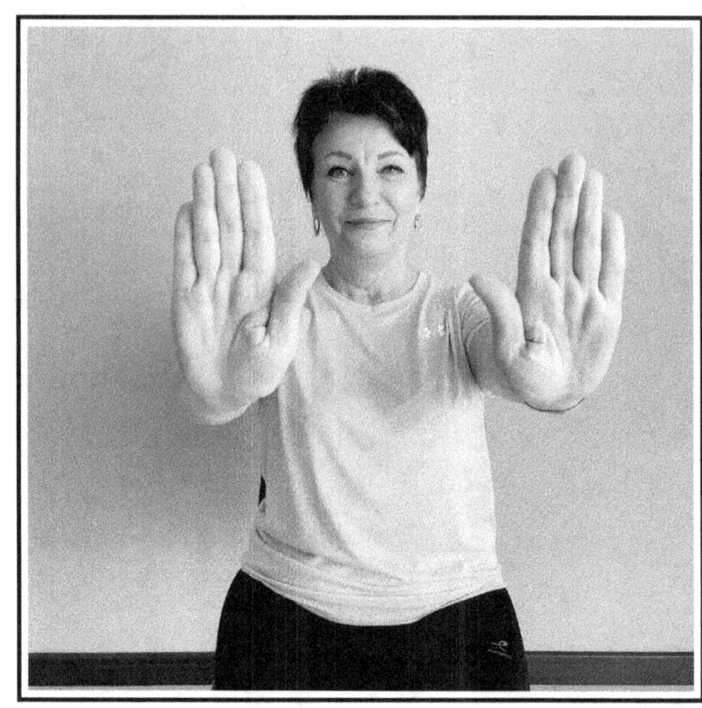

1. Sit tall on the chair and extend your arms out in front of you
2. Keep your fingers straight with palms facing down
3. Inhale, and slowly flex your wrists down
4. Exhale, and extend your wrists up
5. Repeat the movement

- Don't go too fast
- Don't hold the breath
- Don't go to a painful range of motion
- Extend your arms out throughout the whole movement

Fist Circles

This exercise improves your wrist mobility.

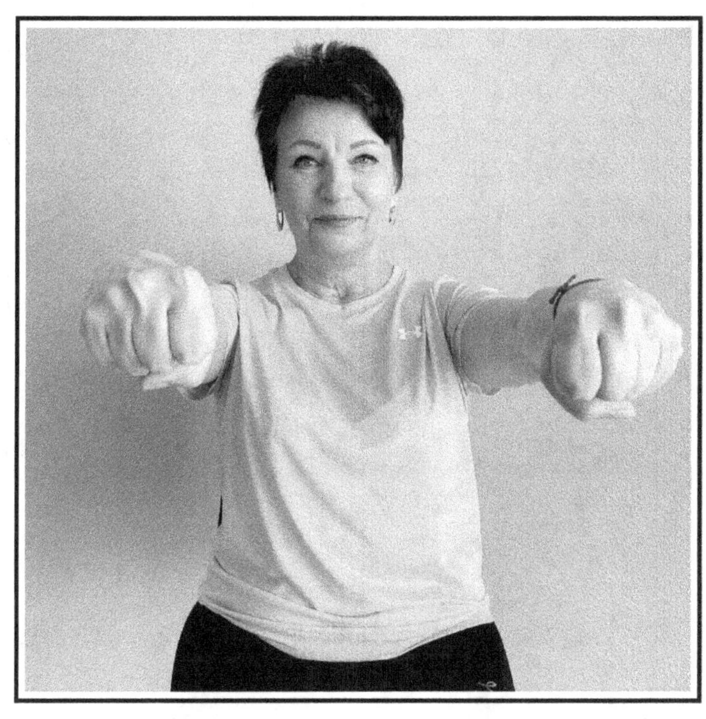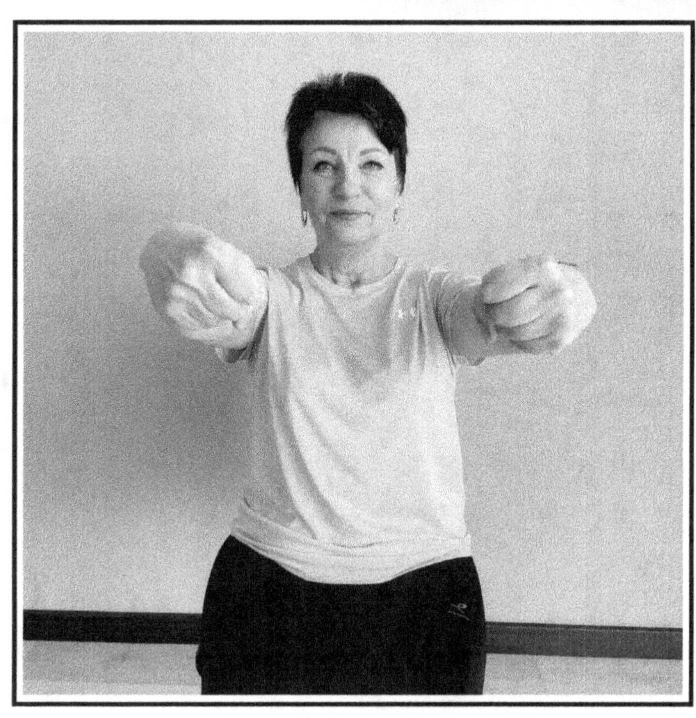

1. Sit tall on the chair and extend your arms out in front of you
2. Keep your hands gently closed
3. Take a deep breath
4. Make two circles with your fists inside, then outside
5. Repeat the movement

SUGGESTED TIPS:

- Don't squeeze your fists too hard
- Don't bend the arms
- Don't go to a painful range of motion
- Keep your arms extended throughout the whole movement

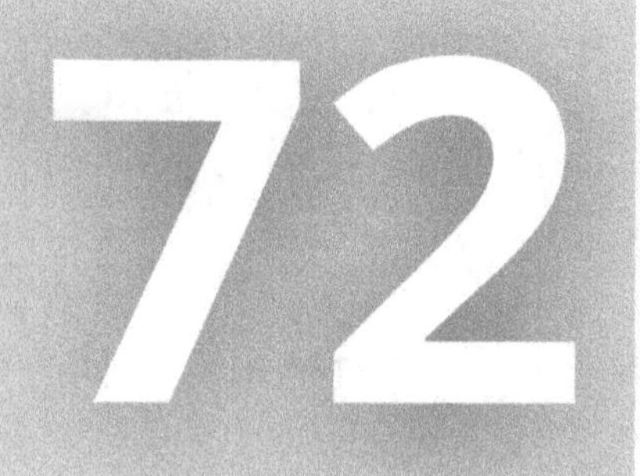

72 Finger Spread

This exercise strengthens your wrist tendons. It gives you a nice stretch in the hands.

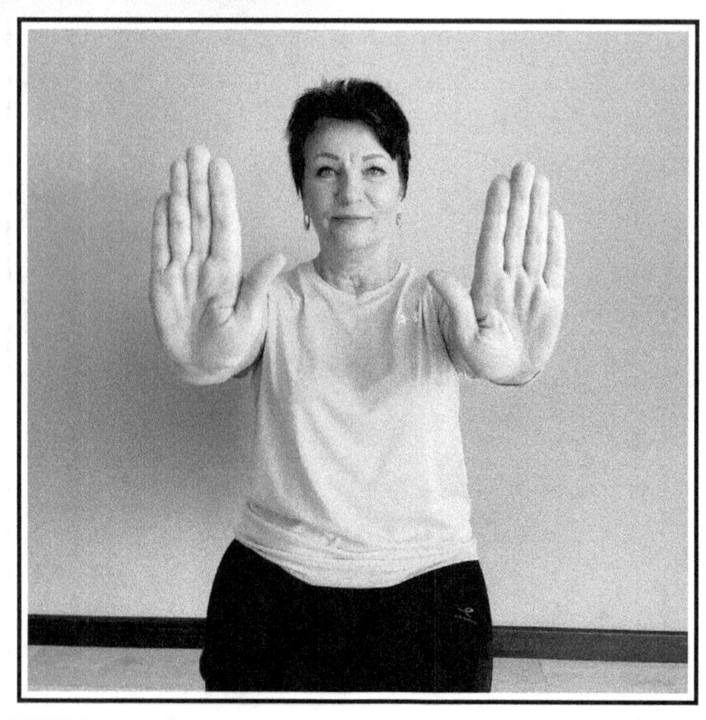 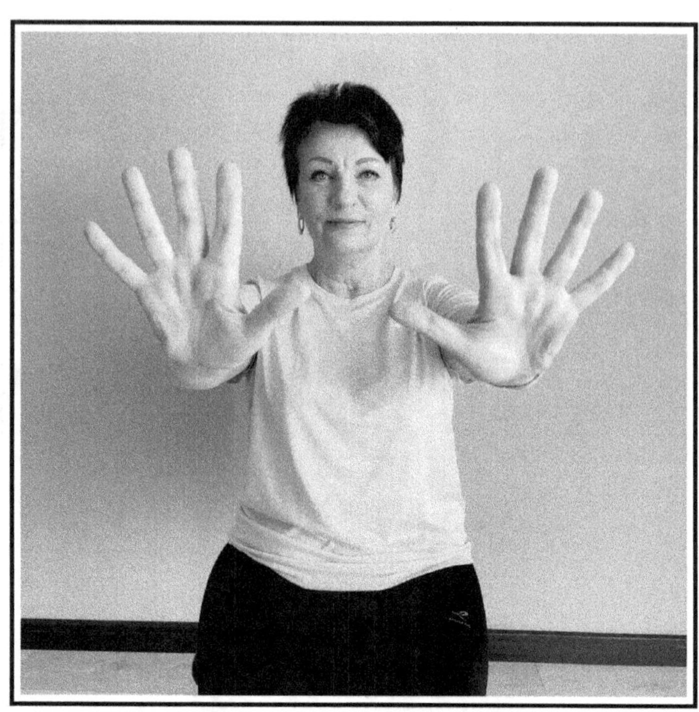

PROCEDURE:

1. Sit tall on the chair and extend your arms out in front of you
2. Put your fingers together and make sure they're pointing toward the ceiling
3. Inhale
4. Spread your fingers as much as you can
5. Close them back again and exhale
6. Repeat the movement

SUGGESTED TIPS:

- Don't hold the breath
- Don't bend the arms
- Don't go to a painful range of motion
- Don't rush with opening and closing your fingers
- Move slowly throughout the exercise

Tuck and Roll

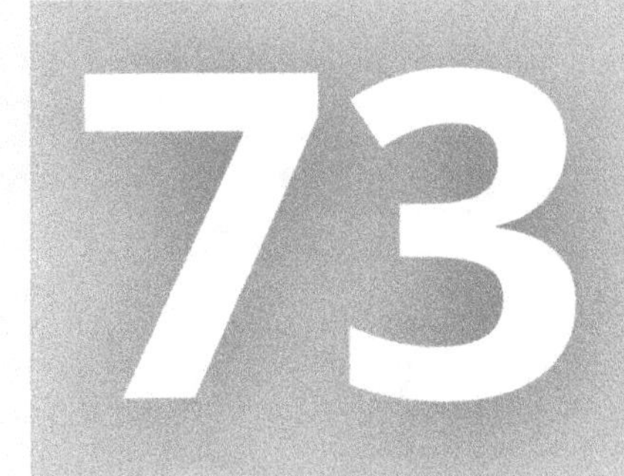

This exercise strengthens your forearm muscles and wrists.

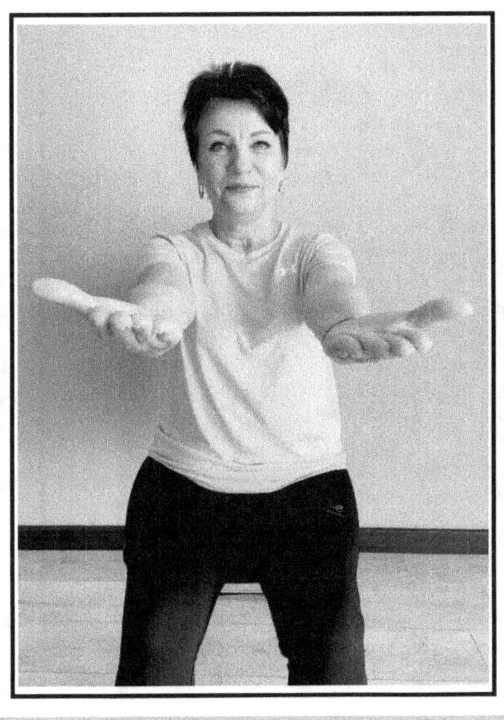 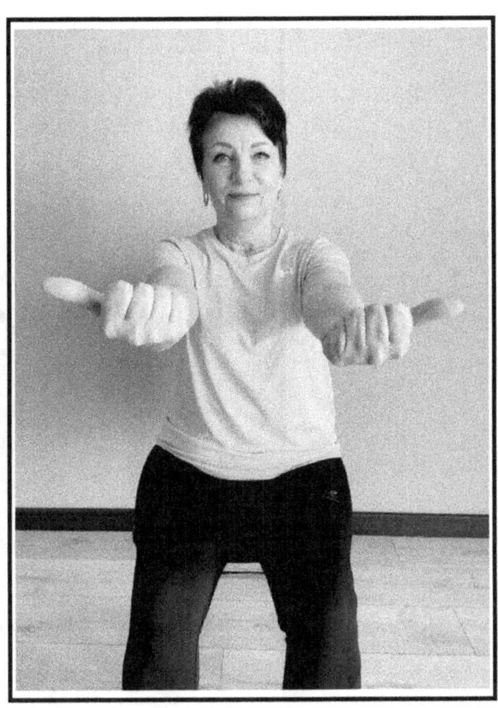 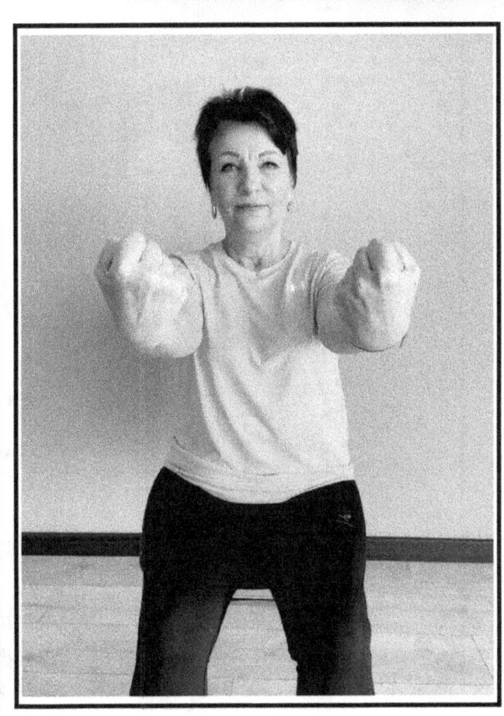

PROCEDURE:

1. Sit tall on the chair
2. Extend your arms out forward
3. Palms should be facing the ceiling
4. Slowly bend the fingers and roll them to a tight fist
5. Release the grip
6. Repeat the movement

SUGGESTED TIPS:

- Don't hold the breath; don't bend the arms
- Don't rush the movement
- Make sure to breathe when doing this exercise
- Inhale at the beginning of the exercise
- Exhale when releasing the fist

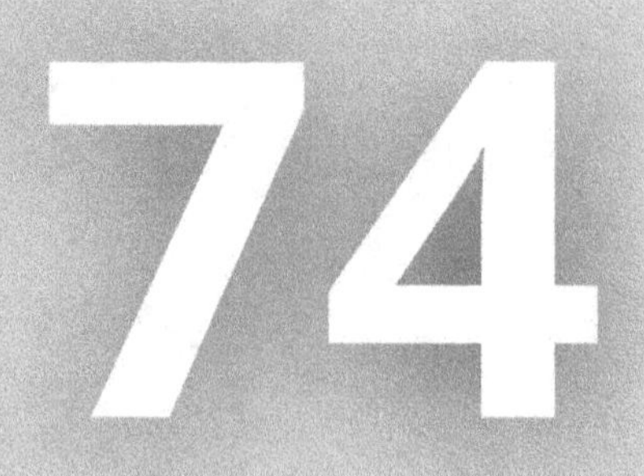

74

Piano Player

This exercise is good for tendon health. It's also a good warm-up exercise for harder wrist exercises.

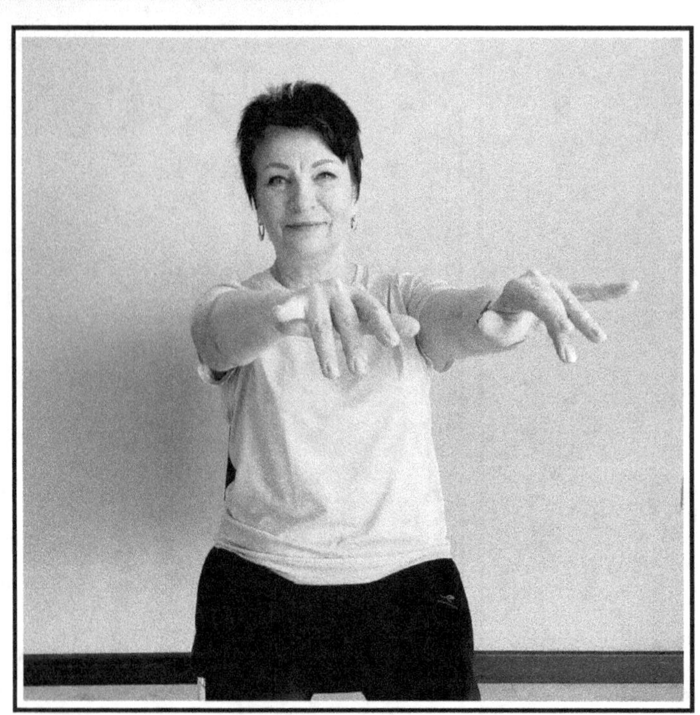 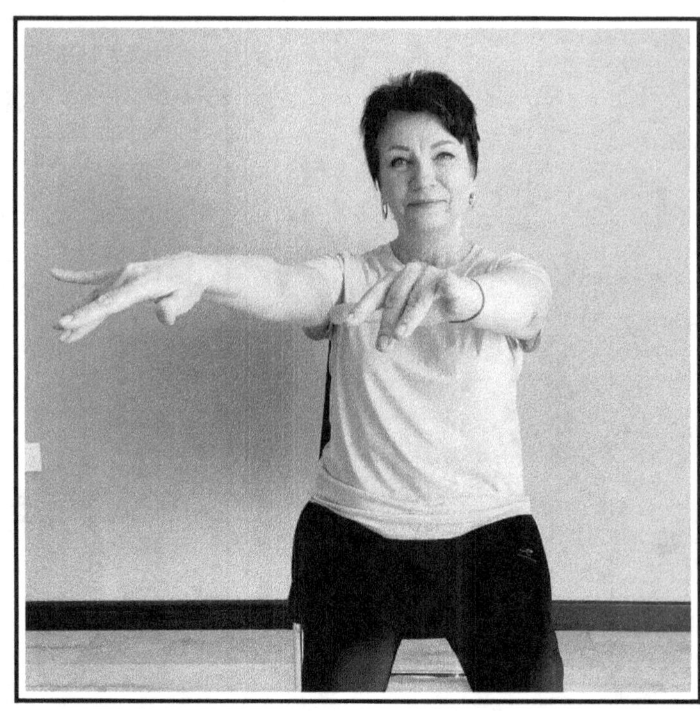

PROCEDURE:

1. Sit tall on the chair
2. Extend your arms out forward
3. Extend your fingers
4. Start moving your fingers up and down like playing a piano and move your hands from side to side

SUGGESTED TIPS:

- This exercise is good for tendon health. It's also a good warm-up exercise for harder wrist exercises.

Close and Open

This exercise activates your forearm muscles.

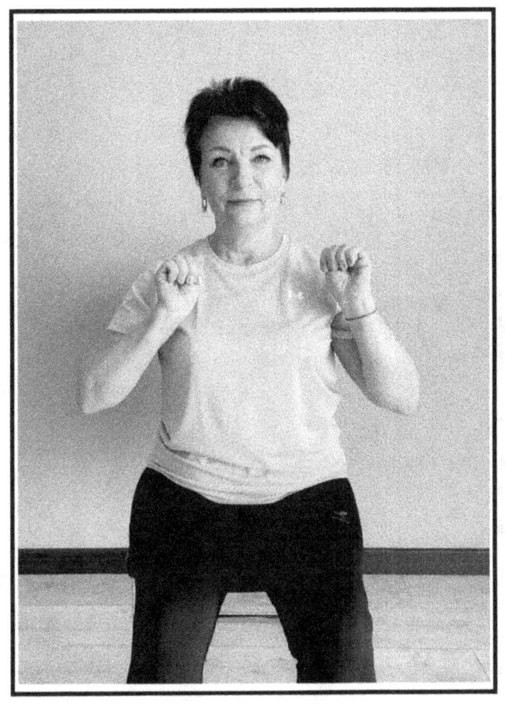
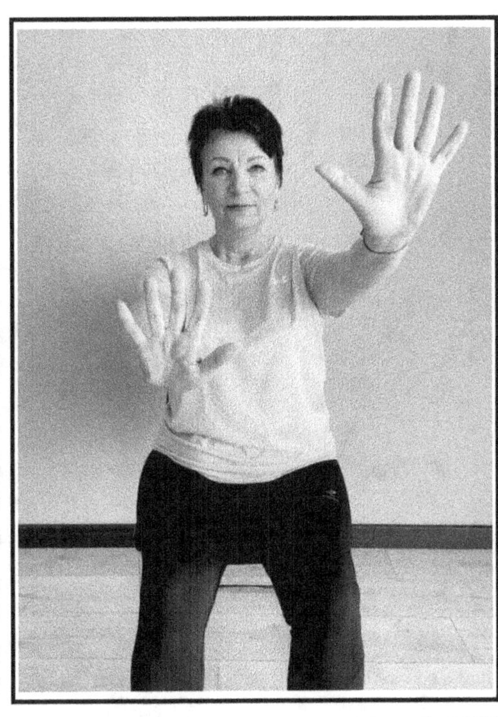
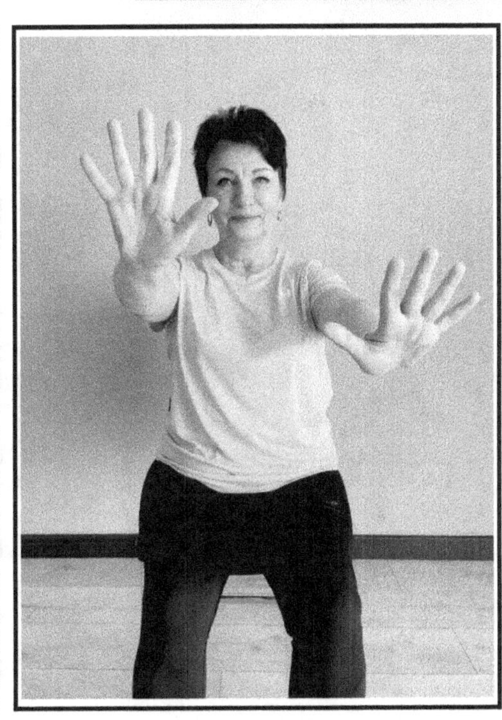

PROCEDURE:

1. Sit tall on the chair
2. Bend your arms and bring your fists to the chest level; inhale
3. Simultaneously, extend your arms out forward and open your hands; exhale
4. Repeat the movement

SUGGESTED TIPS:

- Don't hold the breath
- Don't arch the back
- Don't move too fast
- Relax and breathe throughout this exercise
- Control the pace throughout this exercise

76 Claw (Right, Left)

The exercise activates your forearm muscles and strengthens your wrist tendons.

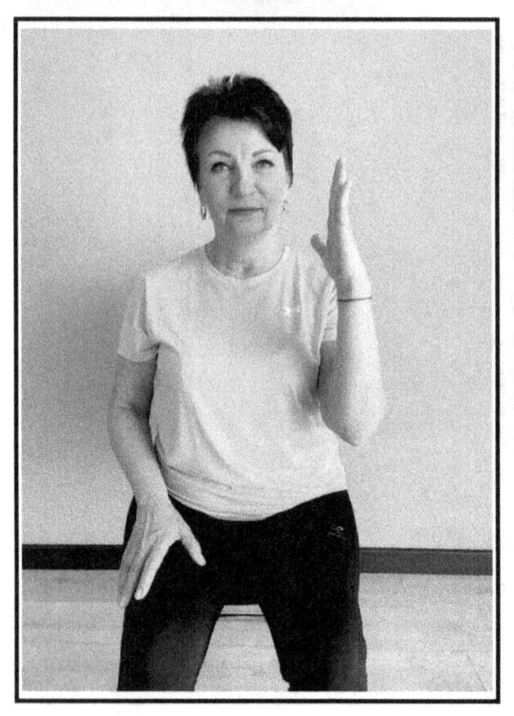 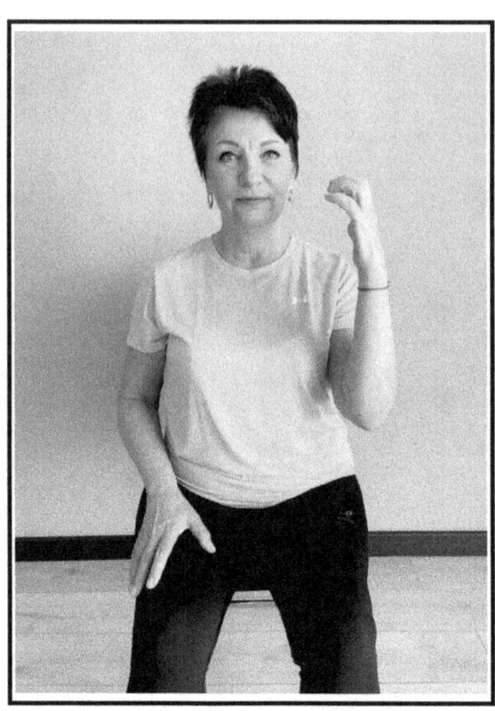 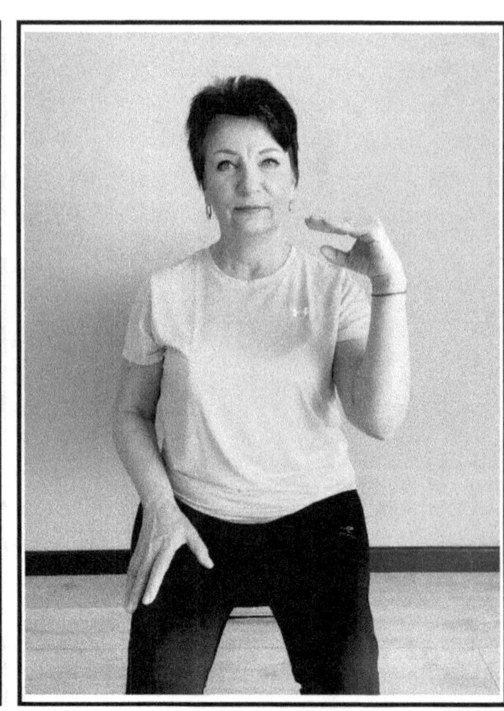

PROCEDURE:

1. Sit tall on the chair
2. Bend your right elbow with fingers facing up
3. Bend your fingers at the knuckles on the right hand
4. Make a claw (think about squeezing a soft ball with your fingers)
5. Repeat the movement
6. Perform the same exercise with the left hand

SUGGESTED TIPS:

- Don't hold the breath
- Don't rush the movement
- Inhale at the start of the movement
- Slowly exhale when beginning to make the claw

Spider Pose

This exercise will stretch your hand and strengthen your fingers.

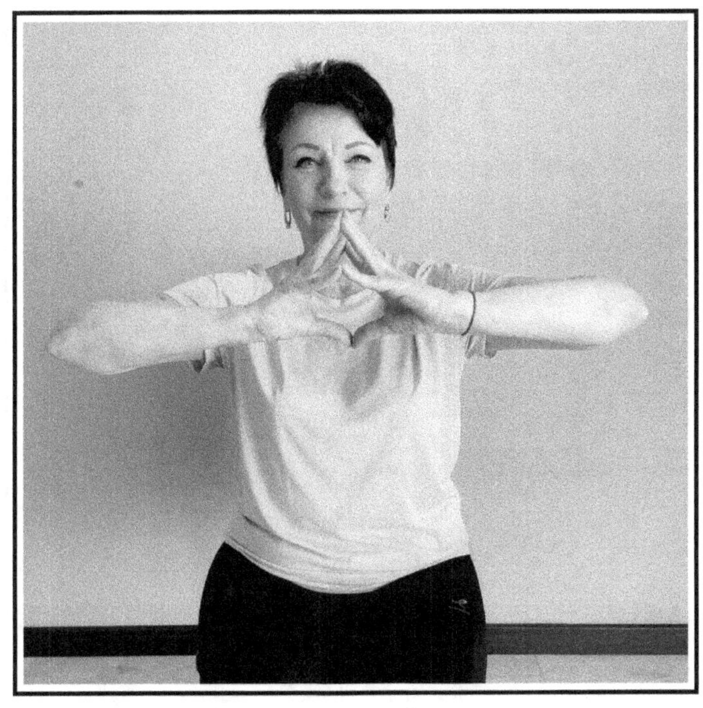

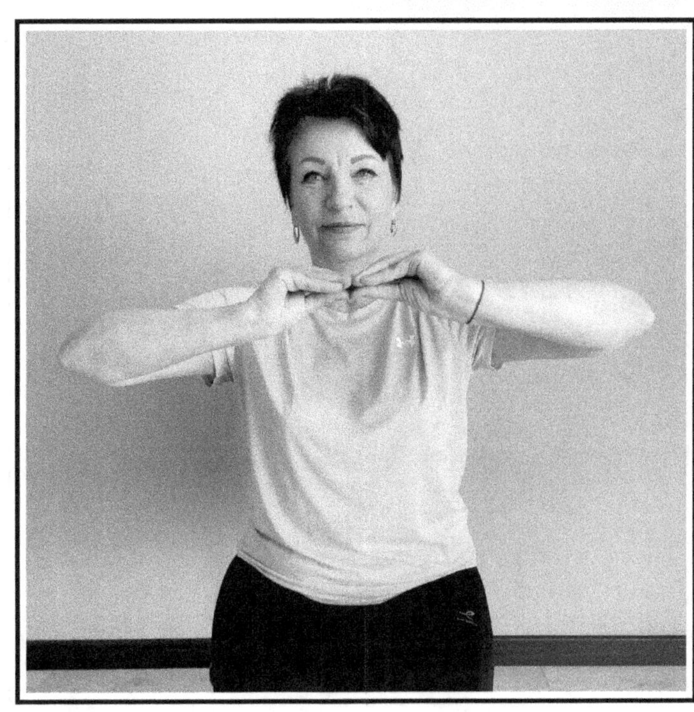

PROCEDURE:

1. Sit tall on the chair
2. Put your elbows to the side
3. Bring the fingertips together
4. Press on the fingertips; let the fingers stretch
5. Curl your fingers down together
6. Repeat the movement

SUGGESTED TIPS:

- Don't close your palms
- Don't extend the elbows
- Don't hold your breath
- Maintain regular breathing throughout this exercise

Finger Stretch (Right, Left)

This exercise is perfect for strengthening your wrist tendons.

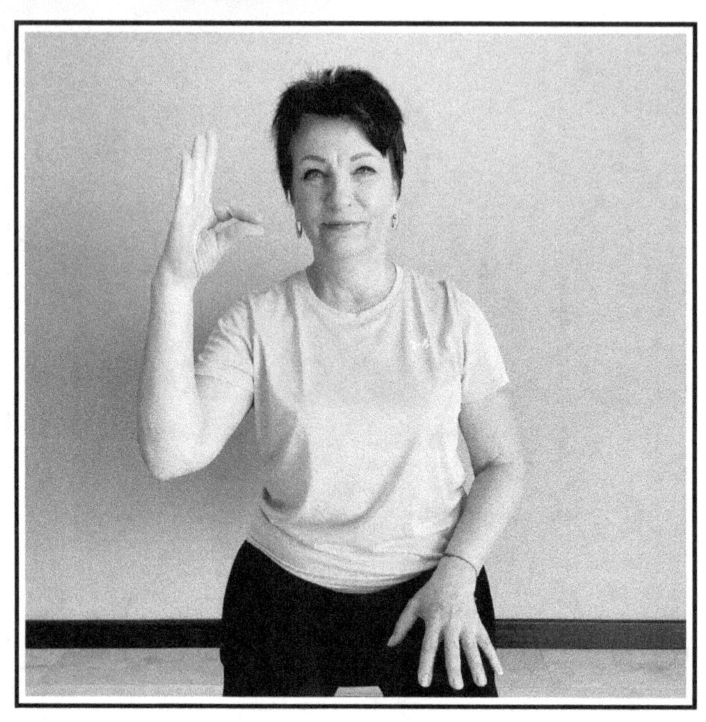 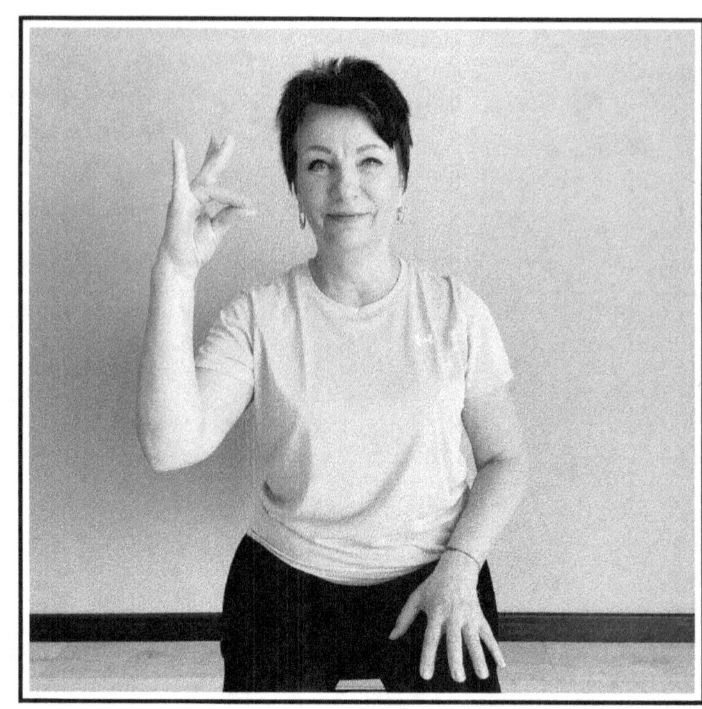

PROCEDURE:

1. Sit tall on the chair
2. Bend your left elbow with fingers facing up
3. Bring your index finger to your thumb and let it stretch; bring it back
4. Bring your middle finger to your thumb and let it stretch; bring it back
5. Bring your ring to your thumb and let it stretch
6. Bring your pinky finger to your thumb and let it stretch; bring it back
7. Bring your thumb under your pinky finger and let it stretch; bring it back
8. Repeat the exercise
9. Perform the same exercise with the right arm

SUGGESTED TIPS:

- Don't hold the breath
- Don't forget to use all fingers
- Maintain regular breathing throughout the exercise
- Make sure to hold each stretch for five seconds

Thumb Tapping

This exercise will strengthen your thumb tendons.

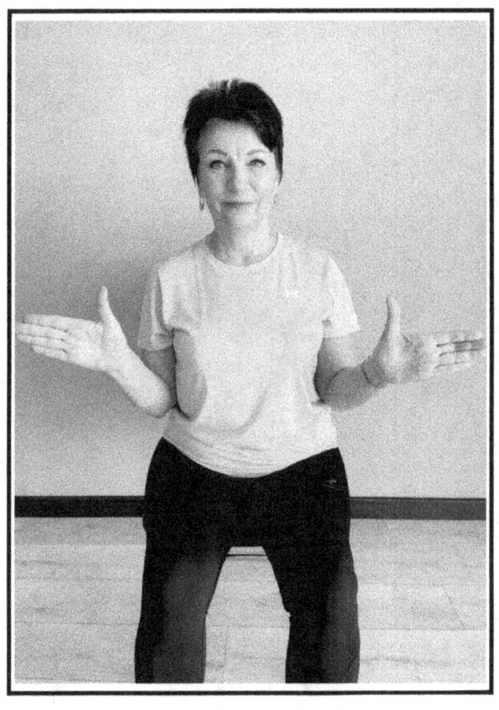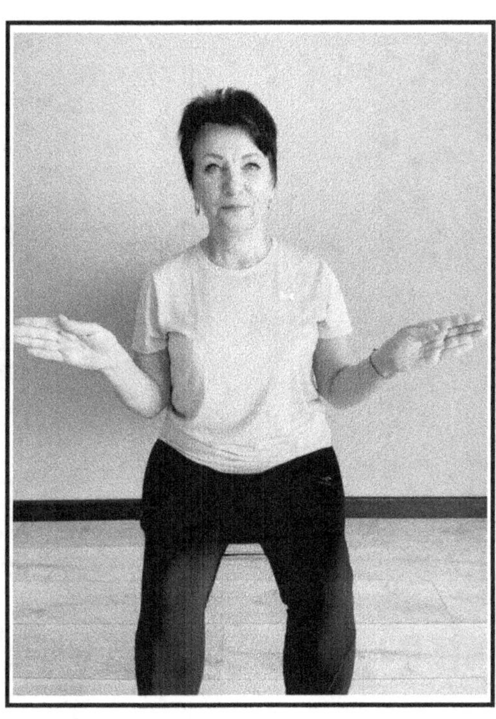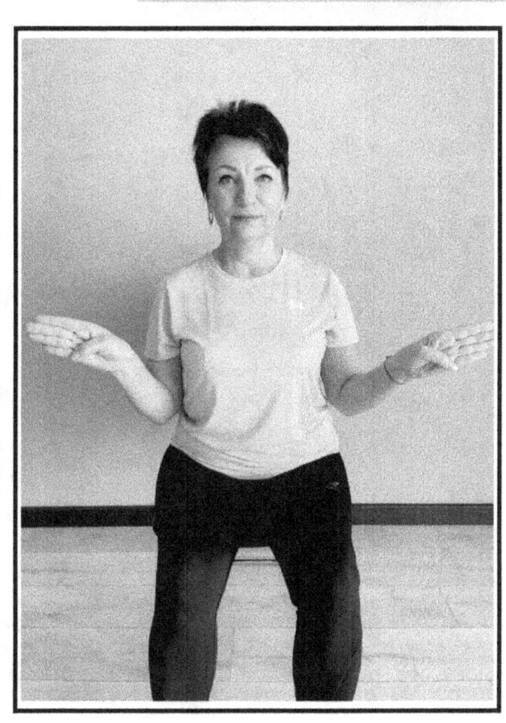

PROCEDURE:

1. Sit tall on the chair
2. Bend your elbows gently
3. Open your palms with your thumbs facing up and the other fingers to the outside
4. Tap your thumb to your index finger three times
5. Tap your thumb to your pinky finger three times
6. Repeat the exercise

SUGGESTED TIPS:

- Don't go too fast
- Don't hold the breath

28-Day Workout Challenge

DAY 1
Hands & Shoulders

WARM-UP
1 - 30 sec
5 - 30 sec
10 - 30/30 sec

MAIN WORKOUT
14 - 40 sec
16 - 40 sec
20 - 40 sec
50 - 40/40 sec
22 - 40/40 sec

STRETCHING
63 - 30/30 sec
67 - 30 sec

DAY 2
Full Body

WARM-UP
6 - 30 sec
4 - 30 sec
9 - 30/30 sec

MAIN WORKOUT
38 - 40 sec
43 - 40 sec
50 - 40/40 sec
54 - 40 sec
19 - 40 sec

STRETCHING
65 - 30 sec
69 - 30 sec

DAY 3
Legs & Hips

WARM-UP
1 - 30 sec
2 - 30 sec
11 - 30 sec

MAIN WORKOUT
24 - 40/40 sec
23 - 40 sec
27 - 40/40 sec
49 - 40 sec
10 - 40/40 sec

STRETCHING
64 - 30/30 sec
62 - 30/30 sec

DAY 4
Full Body

WARM-UP
3 - 30 sec
12 - 30/30 sec
13 - 30/30 sec

MAIN WORKOUT
37 - 40 sec
44 - 40 sec
49 - 40 sec
55 - 40 sec
25 - 40 sec

STRETCHING
68 - 30 sec
65 - 30 sec

DAY 5
Back

WARM-UP
7 - 30 sec
2 - 30 sec
10 - 30/30 sec

MAIN WORKOUT
29 - 40 sec
32 - 40 sec
33 - 40 sec
60 - 40 sec
35 - 40 sec

STRETCHING
66 - 30 sec
69 - 30 sec

DAY 6
Full Body

WARM-UP
3 - 30 sec
8 - 30 sec
9 - 30/30 sec

MAIN WORKOUT
39 - 40 sec
46 - 40 sec
51 - 40 sec
56 - 40 sec
31 - 40 sec

STRETCHING
63 - 30/30 sec
64 - 30/30 sec

Take a 15-30 second break between exercises, depending on how you feel, to allow your body to recover and maintain optimal performance

DAY 7
DAY OFF

DAY 8

Full Body

WARM-UP
2 - 30 sec
12 - 30/30 sec
13 - 30/30 sec

MAIN WORKOUT
40 - 40 sec
45 - 40 sec
52 - 40 sec
57 - 40 sec
23 - 40 sec

STRETCHING
63 - 30/30 sec
67 - 30/30 sec

DAY 9

Back

WARM-UP
1 - 30 sec
3 - 30 sec
11 - 30 sec

MAIN WORKOUT
30 - 40/40 sec
31 - 40 sec
34 - 40 sec
47 - 40 sec
36 - 40 sec

STRETCHING
65 - 30 sec
69 - 30 sec

DAY 10

Full Body

WARM-UP
6 - 30 sec
4 - 30 sec
10 - 30/30 sec

MAIN WORKOUT
41 - 40 sec
47 - 40 sec
53 - 40 sec
58 - 40 sec
33 - 40 sec

STRETCHING
64 - 30/30 sec
62 - 30/30 sec

DAY 11

Hands & Shoulders

WARM-UP
5 - 30 sec
8 - 30 sec
9 - 30/30 sec

MAIN WORKOUT
15 - 40 sec
17 - 40 sec
21 - 40 sec
61 - 40/40 sec
18 - 40 sec

STRETCHING
68 - 30 sec
65 - 30 sec

DAY 12

Full Body

WARM-UP
1 - 30 sec
12 - 30/30 sec
13 - 30/30 sec

MAIN WORKOUT
42 - 40 sec
48 - 40 sec
38 - 40 sec
59 - 40 sec
20 - 40 sec

STRETCHING
66 - 30 sec
69 - 30 sec

DAY 13

Legs & Hips

WARM-UP
2 - 30 sec
7 - 30 sec
11 - 30 sec

MAIN WORKOUT
25 - 40 sec
28 - 40 sec
26 - 40 sec
44 - 40 sec
9 - 40/40 sec

STRETCHING
63 - 30/30 sec
64 - 30/30 sec

Take a 15-30 second break between exercises, depending on how you feel, to allow your body to recover and maintain optimal performance

DAY 14

DAY OFF

DAY 15
Hands & Shoulders

WARM-UP
1 - 30 sec
5 - 30 sec
10 - 30/30 sec

MAIN WORKOUT
14 - 50 sec
16 - 50 sec
20 - 50 sec
50 - 50/50 sec
22 - 50/50 sec
54 - 50 sec

STRETCHING
63 - 30/30 sec
67 - 30 sec

DAY 16
Full Body

WARM-UP
6 - 30 sec
4 - 30 sec
9 - 30/30 sec

MAIN WORKOUT
38 - 50 sec
43 - 50 sec
50 - 50/50 sec
54 - 50 sec
19 - 50 sec
55 - 50 sec

STRETCHING
65 - 30 sec
69 - 30 sec

DAY 17
Legs & Hips

WARM-UP
1 - 30 sec
2 - 30 sec
11 - 30 sec

MAIN WORKOUT
24 - 50/50 sec
23 - 50 sec
27 - 50/50 sec
49 - 50 sec
10 - 50/50 sec
60 - 50 sec

STRETCHING
64 - 30/30 sec
62 - 30/30 sec

DAY 18
Full Body

WARM-UP
3 - 30 sec
12 - 30/30 sec
13 - 30/30 sec

MAIN WORKOUT
37 - 50 sec
44 - 50 sec
49 - 50 sec
55 - 50 sec
25 - 50 sec
57 - 50 sec

STRETCHING
68 - 30 sec
65 - 30 sec

DAY 19
Back

WARM-UP
7 - 30 sec
2 - 30 sec
10 - 30/30 sec

MAIN WORKOUT
29 - 50 sec
32 - 50 sec
33 - 50 sec
60 - 50 sec
35 - 50 sec
58 - 50 sec

STRETCHING
66 - 30 sec
69 - 30 sec

DAY 20
Full Body

WARM-UP
3 - 30 sec
8 - 30 sec
9 - 30/30 sec

MAIN WORKOUT
39 - 50 sec
46 - 50 sec
51 - 50 sec
56 - 50 sec
31 - 50 sec
25 - 59 sec

STRETCHING
63 - 30/30 sec
64 - 30/30 sec

Take a 15-30 second break between exercises, depending on how you feel, to allow your body to recover and maintain optimal performance

DAY 21
DAY OFF

DAY 22
Full Body

WARM-UP
2 - 30 sec
12 - 30/30 sec
13 - 30/30 sec

MAIN WORKOUT
40 - 50 sec
45 - 50 sec
52 - 50 sec
57 - 50 sec
23 - 50 sec
56 - 50 sec

STRETCHING
63 - 30/30 sec
67 - 30/30 sec

DAY 23
Back

WARM-UP
1 - 30 sec
3 - 30 sec
11 - 30 sec

MAIN WORKOUT
30 - 50/50 sec
31 - 50 sec
34 - 50 sec
47 - 50 sec
36 - 50 sec
61 - 50/50 sec

STRETCHING
65 - 30 sec
69 - 30 sec

DAY 24
Full Body

WARM-UP
6 - 30 sec
4 - 30 sec
10 - 30/30 sec

MAIN WORKOUT
41 - 50 sec
47 - 50 sec
53 - 50 sec
58 - 50 sec
33 - 50 sec
54 - 50 sec

STRETCHING
64 - 30/30 sec
62 - 30/30 sec

DAY 25
Hands & Shoulders

WARM-UP
5 - 30 sec
8 - 30 sec
9 - 30/30 sec

MAIN WORKOUT
15 - 50 sec
17 - 50 sec
21 - 50 sec
61 - 50/50 sec
18 - 50 sec
55 - 50 sec

STRETCHING
68 - 30 sec
65 - 30 sec

DAY 26
Full Body

WARM-UP
1 - 30 sec
12 - 30/30 sec
13 - 30/30 sec

MAIN WORKOUT
42 - 50 sec
48 - 50 sec
38 - 50 sec
59 - 50 sec
20 - 50 sec
59 - 50 sec

STRETCHING
66 - 30 sec
69 - 30 sec

DAY 27
Legs & Hips

WARM-UP
2 - 30 sec
7 - 30 sec
11 - 30 sec

MAIN WORKOUT
25 - 50 sec
28 - 50 sec
26 - 50 sec
44 - 50 sec
9 - 50/50 sec
60 - 50 sec

STRETCHING
63 - 30/30 sec
64 - 30/30 sec

Take a 15-30 second break between exercises, depending on how you feel, to allow your body to recover and maintain optimal performance

DAY 28
DAY OFF

28-Day Challenge for Arthritis

28-Day Challenge for Arthritis

DAY 1
70 - 30 sec
76 - 30/30 sec
77 - 30 sec

DAY 2
71 - 30 sec
77 - 30 sec
72 - 30 sec

DAY 3
72 - 30 sec
78 - 30/30 sec
74 - 30 sec

DAY 4
73 - 30 sec
79 - 30 sec
75 - 30 sec

DAY 5
74 - 30 sec
70 - 30 sec
78 - 30/30 sec

DAY 6
75 - 30 sec
71 - 30 sec
73 - 30 sec

DAY 7
DAY OFF

DAY 8
75 - 30 sec
71 - 30 sec
73 - 30 sec

DAY 9
70 - 30 sec
76 - 30/30 sec
77 - 30 sec

DAY 10
71 - 30 sec
77 - 30 sec
72 - 30 sec

DAY 11
72 - 30 sec
78 - 30/30 sec
74 - 30 sec

DAY 12
73 - 30 sec
79 - 30 sec
75 - 30 sec

DAY 13
74 - 30 sec
70 - 30 sec
78 - 30/30 sec

DAY 14
DAY OFF

DAY 15
74 - 40 sec
70 - 40 sec
78 - 40/40 sec

DAY 16
75 - 40 sec
71 - 40 sec
73 - 40 sec

DAY 17
70 - 40 sec
76 - 40/40 sec
77 - 40 sec

DAY 18
71 - 40 sec
77 - 40 sec
72 - 40 sec

DAY 19
72 - 40 sec
78 - 40/40 sec
74 - 40 sec

DAY 20
73 - 40 sec
79 - 40 sec
75 - 40 sec

DAY 21
DAY OFF

DAY 22
73 - 50 sec
79 - 50 sec
75 - 50 sec

DAY 23
74 - 50 sec
70 - 50 sec
78 - 50/50 sec

DAY 24
75 - 50 sec
71 - 50 sec
73 - 50 sec

DAY 25
70 - 50 sec
76 - 50/50 sec
77 - 50 sec

DAY 26
71 - 50 sec
77 - 50 sec
72 - 50 sec

DAY 27
72 - 50 sec
78 - 50/50 sec
74 - 50 sec

DAY 28
DAY OFF

Conclusion

Congratulations, Seniors! You have completed your chair yoga journey. Throughout the book, you've been able to practice the power of yoga from the comfort and support of a chair. Hopefully, you've enjoyed new ways to boost your well-being and vitality with this gentle form of yoga.

We encourage you to continue practicing chair yoga and explore new chair yoga poses and breathing techniques. You can create your own exercise sequences to best fit your personal preferences and adapt to your body and mind. By varying your exercises, you will add depth and richness to your practice which brings a sense of fulfillment.

We want to sincerely thank you for taking this journey with us. We hope that chair yoga continues to be a positive and empowering experience. Approach each practice with a gentle spirit and an open heart, and the yoga will make your days more peaceful, provide you strength, and give you a deep sense of well-being.

Namaste,
FitLife Solutions

References

- Baiera, Vince. (2021, June 15). Benefits of Chair Yoga for Seniors – Reduce Pain and Improve Health. Step 2 Health. https://step2health.com

- Chair Yoga and Why Seated Yoga Poses Are Good for You. (2023, Jan. 1). Lifespan. https://www.lifespan.org

- Chair Yoga Training. (n.d.). Bella Buddha. https://www.bellabuddhayoga.com/chair-yoga-training

- Does Chair Yoga Really Work? (n.d.) Medical News Today. https://www.medicalnewstoday.com/articles/chair-yoga-for-seniors#does-it-work

- Wall Pilates Program: Low Impact Workout Easy for Beginners. (n.d.). Better Me. https://betterme.world